Hospice Volunteer

By Joe Schrantz

(2nd Edition)

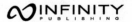 INFINITY PUBLISHING

Copyright © 2003 by Joseph Schrantz

ISBN 978-0-7414-1322-2

Printed in the United States of America

Second Edition

Published January 2012

INFINITY PUBLISHING
1094 New DeHaven Street, Suite 100
West Conshohocken, PA 19428-2713
Toll-free (877) BUY BOOK
Local Phone (610) 941-9999
Fax (610) 941-9959
Info@buybooksontheweb.com
www.buybooksontheweb.com

I dedicate this book to all Hospice volunteers,
their Hospice patients, and their families

The Author

COVER: Author Joe Schrantz (left) looks on as the
spouse of a Hospice patient proudly describes his
photo album.

Contents

Introduction

Why would anyone want to be a hospice volunteer? Good question. Here's how I got started.

Years ago where I worked, there was a lady who, I found out by the grapevine, was a hospice volunteer. A hospice volunteer? You mean, she visited the dying? How depressing! How could anybody do that? I was so impressed by this that I almost literally placed the woman on a pedestal! She was a hospice volunteer! Oh, my God! How could she do it? She therefore must be a very special person!

About this same time, one of my associates at work contracted cancer, and I eventually visited her in the hospice ward of a hospital a week before she died. I had to force myself to go. I didn't go as a volunteer; I felt obligated to go, out of a sense of duty. And once there, I couldn't wait to leave. It was so depressing! I was shocked! Dismayed! Overwhelmed!

Be a hospice volunteer? Not me! Never!

The years passed. I eventually retired and quickly found myself busy with retirement activities. Then one day I saw a feature article in my local newspaper about a retired man who was a hospice volunteer. I read it and was impressed. The man said he received so much more from visiting hospice patients than he gave. Received more than he gave?

Gee, I thought, maybe I could do that. If I could just get over that initial fear, maybe I could do it.

I saved the article, which listed a phone number to call to learn more about becoming a hospice volunteer. Several weeks later I called the number. I soon was undergoing training.

Now, four years later, I can say that being a hospice volunteer is one of the best things that ever happened to me! The man in the newspaper article was absolutely right: the volunteer receives so much more than he gives!

What have I received? When I leave a patient after a visit, I feel 10 feet tall! I overflow with joy! Money can't buy such elation!

Before becoming a hospice volunteer, I was fearful of getting close to the elderly, fearful of entering a nursing home, fearful of being close to the dying. Fearful of death itself.

Now, I don't see death as a monster that's always lurking just around the corner, always following me around. Now, I no longer fear to be near the dying. To the contrary, I find being near the dying a privilege. A sacred privilege! Now, I no longer fear entering a nursing home. I no longer see nursing home residents as scary people to avoid at all costs. To the contrary, I see them as individuals, like you and me, worth getting to know, worth learning to love. Now, I no longer fear getting close to the elderly. I see them as unique individuals, each one precious and worth spending time with.

This kind of maturity can't be bought. It needs to be achieved through giving. But like the man said in the newspaper article: you receive so much more than you give.

Why write a book about some of my experience as a hospice volunteer? Good question. There's the matter of privacy. Hospice volunteers must pledge to respect the privacy of patients. In keeping this pledge, in the following case histories, I have changed or omitted the names of people and places. I have altered certain descriptions. I have omitted dates. My intent is at all times to respect the privacy of the patients I have visited.

The only exception is the case history that deals with Gladys. With her husband's permission, I wrote a book about her (Infinity Publishing, 2002, 820 pages).

Maybe in a small way, writing about my experience will encourage others to give hospice volunteering a try. That newspaper article, after all, prompted *me* to become a hospice volunteer. Maybe this book will encourage *you*.

But, I'm warning you: you'll get hooked. The rewards are too many to count. The joy too rich to contain.

In my four years as a hospice volunteer, I've had perhaps 30 or 40 patients. Here, I write about only 12.

The Author

Mel

I was very nervous and apprehensive as I drove to visit my first hospice patient. Only two weeks earlier I had completed my hospice-volunteer training. In a few minutes I would begin to put into practice what I had learned: how to act when visiting a hospice patient. The main idea, I concluded from the training, boiled down to the following:

- be friendly
- be a good listener
- be of service to the patient and his/her caregiver(s)

Although I knew I wouldn't have difficulty in any of these areas, I was nervous, something like the way I feel when entering a dentist's office. I had been around the elderly and infirm a few times before and always felt uncomfortable. The several times I had been in a nursing home (never as a hospice volunteer), I had wanted out as quickly as possible. It was too depressing. Old people sitting in wheelchairs in hallways: some staring straight ahead as if trying to avoid your gaze; some with their heads sagging forward as if asleep; some looking at you and smiling, as if to invite you to stop and chat. And the smell of excrement, despite attempts by scurrying men and women in white uniforms to tend to the needs of patients.

1

The hospice office had called and told me that my first patient was a man, 81 years old, with lung cancer. His wife didn't want to leave her husband alone; my coming to their home would allow her to go on errands, go to her doctor, go to her hairdresser, go shopping, whatever.

I would be alone with this dying old man. No doubt he had a terrible cough. Would he be able to talk? Would he want to talk? Would he be on oxygen? Would he be coughing up blood? Would I have to help him go to the bathroom? Would he be in diapers? And, heaven forbid, would I be expected to change his diaper?

Why was I doing this? Why did I want to be a hospice volunteer? Was I nuts? Couldn't I find better things to do with my time? What was my problem? How could I be of any use to an old man dying of lung cancer?

I was told to go in the back door, which would be unlocked. Well, that sounded simple enough. I found the house, a modest split-level home. Each house on the block had a mailbox mounted on a post near the street to simplify mail delivery. I opted to pull into the driveway and park near the back door. Straight ahead was a 2 1/2-car garage. No other cars were in the driveway. I looked at my watch. It was a few minutes before 11 o'clock.

The sun was out, but a breeze made the 30-degree temperature seem much colder. My state of apprehension made it feel even colder yet.

I looked down to make sure my brand new hospice volunteer badge was pinned to my sweatshirt. It was. I got out of my car and took a few steps to the back door of what obviously was a big room addition to the house, sort of an enclosed back porch. The addition was surrounded by windows, all of which were closed. A note on the door said, "Come on in, the door's unlocked."

Oh, well, here goes. I opened the door. What the dickens! Cigarette smoke assaulted my nose and lungs. You mean, this man was dying of lung cancer and he was still smoking? Oh, brother! The addictive stranglehold of cigarettes! Gripping right up to the very end of one's life, even though one had lung cancer!

"Hello," I heard a rather muffled voice say off to my right. I turned and looked. There obviously was my patient. He was sitting in a rocking chair and was wearing a heavy plaid jacket and a fur cap with the sides pulled down to keep his ears warm. He had a blanket pulled up around his shoulders. He was smoking a cigarette.

Oh, no! I'm going to have to sit in this smoke-filled room and visit my patient and have to pretend I'm oblivious of the cigarette smoke, which I hate! Oh, boy! This was going to be a long day. And, my poor lungs!

The room was cold. No wonder my patient was dressed so warmly. Apparently he wasn't allowed to smoke in the house proper. Maybe I could open some windows. But then, it was cold outside. I would rather be cold and breathe fresh air. But what about my patient? Could he stand the cold air? But the room was already cold.

"Hi. My name is Joe Schrantz. I'm the hospice volunteer. And you must be Mel."

"Yeah. That's me," he smiled.

He took a long drag on his cigarette, inhaled deeply, and blew the smoke toward me. Then he coughed. It wasn't an ordinary cough, but a deep-down racking of the chest. So this is what a lung cancer cough is like! Boy, it sounds awful! And to think that he's smoking right up to the very end. Oh, well, if he's dying, why give up the habit? He finished his cough by taking out a blue polka dot handkerchief from a pocket, spitting into it, wadding it up, and putting it back into the pocket from whence it came.

I went over to him to shake his hand. It was a limp handshake. But what was I to expect from an old man dying of lung cancer. I sat down in a straight-backed wooden chair opposite him. He had his back to the main part of the house, and about 10 feet separated us.

"They told me I was going to be your first hospice patient and that I would have to break you in," he laughed, bringing up another deep and terrible-sounding cough. He spat into the handkerchief.

Hey, this guy's got a sense of humor. This might be fun after all.

"Yeah, that's right. You're my very first hospice patient. And you get to break me in," I laughed. How could I laugh in a situation like this? I'm in a room full of smoke, which I hate. I'm cooped up with an old man dying of lung cancer. If only I could be some place else, anywhere but in this awful smoke-filled room.

"Well, I'll break you in real good," he laughed again.

As he talked, I studied his face. He was handsome, with brown eyes, but without

4

distinguishing features. Everything was in proper proportion: forehead, nose, cheek bones, mouth, chin.

I wanted to complain about the smoke, but thought I had better wait, at least until I got to know this guy.

I turned my head to the left toward the sound of the back door of the house opening. A woman entered the room and smiled warmly.

"Hi, you must be the hospice volunteer. My name is Catherine. I'm Mel's wife."

"Hi, I'm Joe Schrantz, the hospice volunteer." She limped as she took a few steps toward me. Now what was her problem? Why the limp? She had a kind and compassionate face and a lot of gray hair. She was a few inches shorter than I and had a matronly figure. I thought her to be neither fat nor skinny. I figured she was probably in her midseventies. No way did she look to be as old as her husband. She squeezed my hand warmly.

"My goodness, but it's smoky in here. Would you like a couple of windows open?" she asked.

"Say, that would be nice," I said. I wanted to say that I would kill to have a couple of windows open. She went to a window and raised one.

"Could I go on the other side of the room and open one? That would give some cross ventilation," I said.

"Sure. Mel won't mind. He's dressed warm."

"Yeah, open all the windows you want. I'm dressed good and warm," he smiled.

I wanted to take his advice and open all the windows around the room, but just opened one

5

on the other side to provide some cross ventilation.

"The hospice organization said you could sit with Mel while I go to the doctor," she said. "I don't like to leave him alone. I broke my hip recently in a car accident. That's why I'm limping. I'm supposed to have a bone scan. I'll be leaving in a few minutes. How long can you stay?"

"As long as you want. I'm retired and have all day. I'm at your service." I sat back down, feeling a lot better now that two windows were open. I could already detect a trickle of fresh air coming in.

"Well, nice to have you. Make yourself at home," she said. "I'll go back in the house and finish getting ready and then leave."

"Okay. Nice to meet you, Catherine." I got to my feet as she turned to go back into the house.

"I'm his first hospice patient," Mel said. "I'm supposed to break him in," he laughed.

"Oh, is that right? This is your first hospice patient?"

"Yes, I'm a brand new volunteer. I just took my training a few weeks ago."

"I'll break him in real good," Mel laughed again.

I felt a warm glow. Hey, I like this guy. And I like his wife. This may not be so bad after all, despite the smoke.

"So, tell me about yourself," I said, searching for something to say. I didn't want to start telling him about myself. After all, he was the one who was dying.

He took another drag from his cigarette and blew the smoke toward me again. Oh, well, why worry. The open windows will carry the smoke out eventually.

Mel laughed. "Tell you about myself? Where do I start? I'm eighty-one years old and have lived a long time and have a lot to tell."

"For starters, I'll ask you a few questions. Do you and your wife have children and grandchildren?"

"Do we have children and grandchildren?" he laughed and then coughed. It wasn't the deep-down cough he had done earlier. The blue handkerchief didn't come out. "I'll say we do. She has seven children, and I have two. It's our second marriage. Her first husband died, and my first wife died. And between us we have thirty grandchildren."

"Thirty grandchildren? Wow!" I was going to tell him that my wife and I have 19 grandchildren, but decided not to. I didn't want to start talking about myself.

"And we have ten great-grandchildren," he smiled again.

"Ten great-grandchildren? Holy mackerel!"

The back door opened again and Catherine entered the room.

"I'm leaving now. After I leave, maybe you can help Mel with his breakfast."

"His breakfast?"

"Yes. He sleeps until about ten o'clock. Then the first thing he does is come out here and have a cup of coffee and a couple of cigarettes. I left his breakfast on the counter."

"You don't allow smoking inside the house proper?" I asked.

"No. I don't smoke and don't allow anyone to smoke in the house," she said.

"Sure, I can help him with his breakfast. Oh, I have to move my car so you can get out of the driveway."

I hurried out to my car and parked it on the street and returned to the room.

"Okay. Good-bye, dear, and good-bye, Joe," she said. She pointed a remote control at the garage door, and I saw the door begin to raise. She opened the back door and stepped outside. I watched her walk slowly, limping to the garage, some 25 feet away.

"So, your wife injured her hip in a car accident?"

"Yeah. She was sitting in the back seat by the left door when the car pulled out onto a highway. An oncoming car crashed into the side of the car, right where she was sitting. It really did a number on her hip. She's had surgery to put the hip back together. She's in a lot of pain. I guess she will probably need several more surgeries to correct the problem."

"Oh, boy, that sounds painful. Where did the accident occur?"

"On a highway a little ways west of here. We were in a car with some friends on our way home from a wedding reception."

"Were you driving the car?"

"No. I was in the back seat next to my wife. Her sitting next to the door cushioned the impact for me. I wasn't hurt at all."

8

We paused to watch his wife back their blue Pontiac out of the driveway.

"You haven't had your breakfast yet?" I asked.

"No. I sleep late and come out here and have a cup of coffee and a couple of cigarettes. Then I have my breakfast."

"Are you about ready for your breakfast?" I glanced at my watch. It was almost 11:30.

"Yeah, I guess." He reached over and mashed his cigarette against the side of a floor-stand ash tray practically overflowing with butts.

"Can I help you get up?"

"No, I can make it."

He stood up slowly. He was an inch or two taller than I. He bent over and turned off the electric heater near his chair and removed the blanket from around his shoulders, placing it on the rocker. He turned and began to walk slowly toward the back door of the house. I wanted to tell him to stand up straight, that his posture was terrible.

"Should I close the windows?" I asked.

"No, leave them open. It'll help clear out the smoke."

I went ahead of him and opened the door to the house.

"Can I help you up the steps?" I asked, referring to the three steps leading up to the door.

"No, I can make it okay."

Inside the kitchen, Mel said, "Have a seat. I'll get my breakfast and join you."

I sat down at a dinette table and watched Mel head for the refrigerator.

"Can I help you with your breakfast?"

"No. Catherine leaves everything out for me."

He took a half-gallon carton from the refrigerator and poured some milk over what appeared to be corn flakes. He brought the bowl and a small plate bearing a piece of jam-covered toast to the table.

"Can I get you something to drink? A cup of coffee, maybe?" I asked.

"All right. The coffee's over there, and the cups are in the cupboard there."

I was glad to have something to do and got his coffee for him and sat down opposite him.

"So you have a late breakfast?"

"Yeah. I sleep late. What the heck, I'm dying anyway. Why rush to get up early and have breakfast?" he coughed. He brought out the blue handkerchief and spat into it.

"Say, I think I'll go out to my car and bring my lunch in and eat with you."

Minutes later I was sitting down opposite Mel and pouring myself a cup of hot tea from my Thermos. "I fixed myself a peanut butter and honey sandwich."

"You didn't need to bring your lunch. We've got a lot of food here. You could just help yourself."

"Hey, I like your house." I glanced around. The kitchen and living room were one large room comprising the main floor of the house. There seemed to be religious artifacts everywhere: pictures and small statues of Jesus and Mary.

"How long have you had lung cancer, Mel?" I

took a bite of my sandwich and watched him mouth a spoonful of cereal.

"I was diagnosed with lung cancer about six months ago."

"And, you were just put on hospice recently?"

"Yeah."

"And, I suppose you've been given six months to live?" I couldn't believe I had asked that question.

"Actually, my doctor said he expects me to die in four more months."

"Four more months?"

"Yeah. He said I could go anytime before that, but four months at the latest."

"How do you feel about that?"

"I feel good. I've lived a full life. I have no complaints. I'm dying. We're all dying. Some of us are just dying sooner than others."

"Gee, you have a healthy outlook on the situation, don't you?"

"Yeah. I'll be glad to die. What the heck, I'm eighty-one years old. I don't want to live forever. I'm old. I've got cancer. I'm going to die. I'm ready—"

A cough cut off his words. And then another cough, and another. I wanted to help him, but I didn't know what to do. He spat into the handkerchief several times.

When he stopped coughing, I watched him get up. His cereal had hardly been touched. And only one bite had been taken out of his toast.

"I'm going out on the back porch and have another smoke."

"Is there anything I can do for you?" I picked up my cup of tea and my sandwich and followed him.

"No. I'm fine."

"You didn't eat much breakfast."

"That's all I want. I'm not that hungry. I'd rather smoke."

We took our seats again in the back room, Mel with his back to the house and me in the chair facing him. With the two windows still open, the air in the room smelled much better than before, yet the stale odor of cigarette smoke still lingered.

"So, how long have you and Catherine been married?"

"Thirty-one years," Mel said, lighting a cigarette with a lighter. He snapped the lid shut on the lighter and blew smoke toward me. He wrapped the blanket around his shoulders.

We were interrupted by a car in the driveway.

"It looks like Catherine is back," I commented.

She stopped her car in the driveway and entered the back room.

"Hello, dear, I'm back," she smiled. "Hello, Joe. How did things go?"

"Everything went fine. Mel's breaking me in real good. He had his breakfast. That is, he ate part of his breakfast. He said he wasn't very hungry."

"He doesn't eat much breakfast."

"He just took a couple of spoons of cereal and I think only one bite of his toast, and that's it. Then he wanted to come back out here and smoke some more."

"Yes, that's what he does. Oh, well. What can I do?"

"Well, Mel. Listen, you did a great job breaking me in," I laughed. I went over to Mel to shake his hand. "I enjoyed meeting you and talking with you."

I turned to Catherine. "When would you like for me to come back? I'm retired and pretty well free to come back whenever you want. And I live nearby."

"Could you come back next Wednesday? I have another doctor's appointment."

"Sure. Same time? Eleven o'clock?"

"Yes. Make it eleven o'clock. Mel sleeps late and has a late breakfast."

"Okay. Sounds good. I'll see you next Wednesday."

"Oh, before you go, would you mind going out to the mailbox and bringing in the mail?" Catherine asked.

"I'd love to."

I was only too happy to bring in the mail for them. With her limp, it was difficult for her to walk to the mailbox, and with Mel's cancer, all but impossible for him.

Visit 2

At a few minutes before 11 o'clock I parked in the street, making sure I stayed sufficiently away from the mailbox to allow access by the mail car driver. I went around to the back door and entered the room addition. It was practically a repeat of the week before: Mel was sitting in his rocker with his hat on and the flaps pulled down over his ears and with a blanket wrapped around his shoulders. The outdoor temperature was in the 30's, and it didn't feel much warmer than that in the room, which was again filled with smoke.

"Hi, Mel. Boy, is it smoky in here! Would you mind if I opened a few windows?"

"Hi, Joe. Yeah, it is smoky in here. Go ahead and open all the windows you want."

This time I opened two windows on each side of the room. The smell of smoke was repulsive. How could anyone be addicted to inhaling that ghastly stuff? I couldn't fathom it.

"So how's it going, Mel?"

He did one of his deep, terrible-sounding coughs and spat into his blue polka dot handkerchief before he replied.

"About as good as could be expected under the circumstances. And how about yourself?" he smiled. He took a drag from his cigarette and blew the smoke in my direction.

"I'm doing great. After you broke me in last week, I feel like a real pro as a hospice volunteer," I laughed. "You can break me in a little more this week, Mel. Okay? But be gentle!"

Mel joined me in my laughter and coughed again.

I quickly found out that Mel once again had not had his breakfast. He had slept late and was again filling himself with nicotine before he had his bowl of cereal and piece of jam toast.

"I like this room addition. Did you build it, Mel?"

"I helped a son-in-law build it."

I looked around, studying the slanted roof rafters and the electrical conduits, which had obviously been professionally installed.

"I really like it. A professional job."

"Thanks."

Minutes later I followed Mel into the kitchen. We sat down at the table and I began to watch him eat his cereal. Suddenly I remembered.

"Hey, Mel. I just remembered something. I brought you a piece of Greek pastry. I left it out in the car. Wait a minute and I'll get it for you."

I hurried out to my car. I unwrapped the pastry and put it on a plate from a cupboard and set it in front of Mel next to his jam toast.

"I think it's called 'baklava,' or something like that. I bought it at a little store in my wife's cousin's neighborhood. My wife and I went there yesterday. It's the neatest store. It's got the best darn produce. And they sell this Greek pastry. I think you'll like it. I had a piece this morning and I loved it."

Mel mashed off a tip of the pastry with his spoon and tasted it. Without commenting about it, he took another bite, and then another.

"You like it, huh, Mel?"

"Yeah, it's all right."

He kept eating it and minutes later it was gone. I sipped at a cup of tea from my Thermos and ate my peanut butter and honey sandwich as he ate.

"Boy, I'll have to bring you another piece next time I come over. You really liked it, huh?"

"Yeah, it was all right."

Mel got up and headed for the back porch to smoke. He had taken only a couple of spoonfuls of cereal, and he hadn't touched his jam toast.

Back in our seats on the porch, Mel lit another cigarette, snapping shut the lid to his cigarette lighter with a metallic clink.

"Now, tell me some more about yourself. How about starting from the beginning," I said.

"I was born in Montana, not too far from Helena. When I was about seven years old, my dad died, and my mother couldn't take care of us. There were five of us children. She farmed us out to various places. I and my younger sister were put in an orphanage."

"How long did you stay at the orphanage?"

"Until I graduated from high school."

"You mean, all that time, from when you were seven until you graduated from high school, you were at an orphanage?"

"Yeah."

"Oh, my golly! So you were there for about ten years?"

"Something like that."

"Gee. In other words, you were raised at that orphanage. Did you ever see your mother again?"

"I went to see her after I left the orphanage. I went to work for a while, and with World War II getting started about then, I joined the service— the Army Air Corps, as it was called then."

"No kidding! The Army Air Corps. Did you become a pilot?"

"No. I washed out of flight school. I was doing

16

my solo flight at Luke Field outside of Phoenix, and I made a terrible landing. My plane bounced up and down on the runway something awful. My flight instructor washed me out. Then I was sent to gunnery school."

"I'll be darned! I was born and raised in Phoenix. I grew up there before and during World War II. My stepfather worked at Luke Field and took me there to spend the day once. I was really thrilled to see all those AT-6's and P-40's. And one day in Phoenix at the time, when I was in the eighth grade, I was having trouble catching on to taking the square root of a number. So my teacher, a feisty little nun, had one of the smart boys in class take me outside and teach me square root. So while we were sitting on the steps of the school, all of a sudden a flight of about seven P-40's peeled off individually into a dive and then pulled up. The last P-40 plowed smack into a two-winger Steerman trainer. The impact tore the Steerman into a million pieces, and the P-40 went into a dive and crashed. The instructor and student in the Steerman were killed outright, but the instructor and student in the P-40 bailed out and survived. That was quite an experience seeing that mid-air collision."

"So you actually saw that happen?" He coughed again.

"Yeah. During World War II, Phoenix had half a dozen airports in operation for training military pilots."

Mel coughed again. This one was especially bad. If only I could do something for him.

"So, tell me, Mel, then you went to gunnery school. What happened next?"

"I was assigned to a squadron of B-25's and was a tail gunner."

"You were a tail gunner on a B-25? No fooling?"

"Yeah. My squadron was assigned to the South Pacific."

"What kind of missions did your squadron fly? Dropping bombs?"

"No. We went on strafing missions. We shot up whatever we saw on the ground on enemy bases. Buildings, trucks, planes, whatever we saw down there, we shot at it."

"So as the tail gunner, while your plane was strafing things on the ground, what were you doing?"

"Keeping my eye out for enemy aircraft."

"Did you ever see any? And did you ever shoot at any?"

"Yeah, I saw quite a few. And I shot at them plenty!"

"Did you get credit for destroying any enemy planes in the air?"

"Yeah, I got a couple of them."

"Boy, is that exciting. Did you ever have any close calls?"

"I sure did. Our plane was shot at a lot. About half a dozen times or more our plane came back to base shot up pretty badly."

"Holy mackerel! How many missions did you fly?"

"Thirty-seven."

"Thirty-seven missions! Wow!"

Mel coughed again and choked back his tears.

"I was to have gone on my thirty-eighth mission but I told my commanding officer I just couldn't do it, that I was a basket case, just too full of fatigue. And it was on that thirty-eighth mission that our plane was shot down. The entire crew was killed."

"Oh, my God! Who took your place as tail gunner on that flight?"

Mel choked back his tears again.

"It was a young fellow fresh from the states. A real clean-cut looking guy. It was his first mission in a war zone."

"What brought the plane down?"

"It was hit by antiaircraft fire and crashed over the Philippines."

"Oh, my God! Were you ever lucky not to have been on that thirty-eighth flight!"

Mel wiped at his tears with his bare hands.

"It was my fault that that young fellow got killed. I should have gone on that flight. But I just couldn't. I was all stressed out."

"That's easy to understand, Mel. You were completely justified to tell your commanding officer you couldn't go. Then, did you start making flights on another B-25?"

"No. I was sent back to the states for some R and R. Then I was assigned to an air base in Texas as a gunnery instructor until the war ended."

"You really had an exciting experience in the war, didn't you?"

"Yeah."

Mel wiped at his tears again.

"If only I would have gone on that thirty-eighth mission, that new fellow wouldn't have got killed."

"Yeah, but then you would have been killed, Mel. And I wouldn't be sitting here asking you questions. You couldn't help it. You had gone on thirty-seven missions and you just plain needed a rest. It wasn't your fault that your plane went down. You didn't do anything wrong, Mel."

He wiped at his tears again and then went through a long series of awful-sounding coughs.

The door to the back room opened and I turned to see an attractive young lady entering.

"Hi, Mel. How are you doing today?" she asked.

"Hi, Peggy. I'm doing okay."

"Hi. My name is Joe Schrantz, and I'm a hospice volunteer just chatting with Mel," I said, standing up.

"Hi, Joe. Nice to meet you. I'm the hospice nurse. Well, come on inside, Mel, and I'll check your vitals," she said.

I followed them into the kitchen. Mel sat down at the table.

"Would you mind if I hung around a bit and watched?" I smiled.

"Sure, stick around. Have a seat," Mel said. "He's a new hospice volunteer, and I'm breaking him in," he laughed, bringing on another cough.

I looked on fascinated as Peggy took his pulse, blood pressure, and listened to his breathing.

"Mel, you're about the same as you were last

week," Peggy said. "Have you been taking your medicine and eating good?"

"You bet. I learned way back in the service that you don't dare disobey the orders of a nurse. Especially such a pretty one as you," Mel laughed.

"Mel told me he's going to lick this lung cancer," I told Peggy. "Right, Mel?"

"Yeah. The doctor told me I won't be around much longer. But I'm going to fool everybody. I'm going to be around a lot longer than they think." He gave me a wink and smiled, breaking into another cough.

"That's the right attitude, Mel. You just keep following my orders: take your medicine and eat your meals, and you just might prove the doctor wrong after all," Peggy smiled.

We heard a car pull into the driveway. I stood up and looked out and saw it was Catherine's car. She was back from the hair dresser's. I went to open the door of the back room for her.

"Hi, Catherine. Hey, would you just look at that new hair-do! Boy, you look like a movie star now!" I said.

"Ha. That'll be the day," she laughed. "How's Mel doing?"

"Just fine. Peggy, the nurse, is in the kitchen with him, taking his vitals."

I went back into the kitchen with Catherine. She kissed her husband on the cheek and greeted Peggy.

"Well, listen, I think I'll be shoving off," I said. "When would you like me to come back?" I asked Catherine.

"How about next Wednesday again. Same time. About eleven o'clock. It'll give me a chance to get out of the house again."

"Next Wednesday it'll be. Same time, same station," I laughed.

"Oh, could you bring in the mail again before you leave?" Catherine smiled.

"You bet I could!"

Visit 3

A week later Catherine called and said she wouldn't be needing me that week. Several weeks went by before she called again and asked me to come over so she could go on another errand. This time the back room addition didn't seem as cold when I opened the windows to let out the smoke. Catherine left shortly after I arrived—off to another doctor's appointment. I again chatted with Mel while he smoked his prebreakfast cigarettes.

While Mel was eating breakfast he said, "I've got a job for you today."

"You have a job for me? Great, Mel. I'm here to help. What can I do for you?"

"I want you to help me get some of my bookkeeping in order so Catherine won't have to do it after I'm gone."

"I'll be only too happy to help." What was this? Help him get his bookkeeping in order?

"You mean, like, helping you pay some bills, maybe write a few checks or something like that?"

"Yeah, maybe a little of that. But I mainly

want you to help me make sure all my personal stuff is in order: my insurance, my funeral plans, and all that." Mel took a bite of toast and coughed.

"Sounds good, Mel. I'll help in any way I can."

It wasn't that I didn't want to help Mel in these personal areas, it was just that I didn't think it appropriate. Catherine should help him so she would be familiar with everything when Mel dies. But I didn't know how to tell this to Mel.

"Well, come on downstairs and let's get to work," Mel said.

He led me down a flight of stairs to the lower split level, which he called a basement.

"Have a seat," Mel told me. "I'll see if I can find the stuff I'm looking for."

I sat down in an upholstered chair near a lamp and watched Mel riffle through the drawers of a desk.

"Now, where did I put all that stuff?" he said, going through drawer after drawer, sifting through various papers. I got the impression that Mel either had misplaced whatever it was he was looking for, or that his cancer had hacked away at his attention span, making it impossible for him to complete the detailed task at hand.

Finally I told him, "Mel, I have a good idea. How about if you ask Catherine to help you find what you're looking for and then perhaps I can help you with it on my next visit. Or maybe Catherine could help you with it."

"That's a good idea. I think you're right. I'll ask Catherine to help me find the stuff."

We went back upstairs and took our seats in

the room addition.

"Tell me about your first marriage," I said.

"My first wife's name was Ann. We got married while I was in the service. You know, when I got married—" Mel coughed and paused to collect his thoughts. Then he sounded almost apologetic. "When I got married the first time, I didn't know anything at all about—about what a husband was supposed to do." He wiped away a few tears and coughed again.

"You and Ann had two children?"

"Yeah. Two children. Then it wasn't long after the war when she contracted cancer and died."

"I'm so sorry, Mel. Now tell me about meeting Catherine."

"Not too many years later I met Catherine. Her husband had died and had left her with seven children. Well, we got married and made a home for her seven kids and for my two children."

"You and Catherine never had any children of your own?"

"No." He coughed again.

"Say," Mel said, "I sure would like to meet all of the hospice staff. I've met you, and Peggy, the nurse, and the social worker. You know what. I'd like to go over to the hospice office and meet all the rest of the staff."

"You would?"

"Yeah. This hospice organization is really helping me, and I'd like to meet everyone."

"Well, listen. When I get home today, I'll call the hospice office and see if I can take you over there next week. Okay?"

"Okay. I'd like that a lot."

Mel launched into another racking cough, and I started looking around the room. My eyes came to rest on a portable Norelco electric shaver.

"Do you use that shaver?" I asked Mel after he wiped his mouth with his polka dot handkerchief.

"I haven't been using it lately. It hasn't been working very good. I have another one in the bathroom that plugs in that I've been using."

"Mind if I take a look at this one? Maybe I can fix it for you. I have a Norelco at home, too, but it's of the plug-in kind."

I took the shaver to a round table off to my right and sat down in another chair and began to disassemble it. I took out the rotary cutters and blew them off to clean them and reassembled them, making a point to put each cutter into a different mating receptacle. That was the way I cleaned mine at home every other day or so. Then I turned on the shaver.

"It sounds good to me, Mel. Would you like to give it a try?"

"Sure."

I took the shaver to Mel and he turned it on and brought it to his face.

"I'll be darned. It's working good. What did you do to it?"

"Just took it apart and cleaned it."

"Well, great. Now I can use it again. It's always been my favorite."

"It really is a nice one. I think it's the deluxe Norelco model. It costs a lot more than the plug-in model I have at home."

About this time Catherine returned.

"Joe fixed my shaver," he told her.

"He did? Well for heaven's sake! I tried to fix it for him but didn't have any luck. What did you do to it?"

"I just took it apart and cleaned the little cutters and made a point of putting each cutter into a different receptacle. That's what I always do to mine at home," I boasted.

"You did? I thought you were always supposed to keep each cutter in the same receptacle," she said.

"Well, I don't know if you're supposed to or not, but at home I always rotate mine when I clean them and put them back together. And my shaver always works great."

"I thought sure I read in the directions that it specifically says to keep each cutter in the same receptacle," she frowned.

"Well, whatever he did to it, it sure works a lot better than it did," Mel said.

Before I ended my visit, I went to the mailbox and brought in their mail.

Visit 4

As I promised Mel, I called the hospice office when I got home, and I was given approval to bring Mel over to meet the staff. I was told that this had never been done before, but that none of the staff had any objection. I was assured that a wheelchair was available just inside the door of the hospice building, and that I could put Mel in the wheelchair and take him to the second floor in the elevator and wheel him down the hallway to the office.

I backed my car into the driveway, and minutes later I had Mel in the front passenger seat. From Mel's house to the hospice office was only about a mile or so. I stopped my car near the front door and assisted Mel out of the car. I suggested that he wait for me at the curb until I parked my car, maybe a hundred feet away. But when I returned to Mel, he had already gone inside. I was surprised. I didn't think he could open that heavy door by himself.

I found the wheelchair under the stairs, right where I was told it would be, and had Mel sit down in it. I wheeled him into the elevator and went to the second floor and pushed him down a long corridor to the hospice office.

Minutes later I had Mel in a conference room, where the hospice staff was about to assemble for its weekly noon meeting. They typically would gather around a big round table and eat sack lunches as they talked. The last person to enter the room closed the door and sat down. There were about 10 people sitting around the table, including the hospice director, chaplain, several nurses, and the hospice accountant. I occupied a place at the table, and Mel sat in the wheelchair next to me.

"Joe, would you like to introduce your guest," the hospice director, said.

"Certainly. This is Mel, whom I have been visiting now for several weeks. Mel is my very first hospice patient, and he has the somewhat dubious privilege of breaking me in as a volunteer." I paused to laugh.

"I'm breaking him in real good," Mel interrupted. And then he launched into a monologue that went on and on and on. He told:

- how he was breaking me in
- how much he liked the hospice people he had met so far
- how glad he was to get to meet the staff
- how he was going to whip his lung cancer and live at least for another year
- how he had been raised in an orphanage
- how he had married two times
- how he and Catherine raised nine children between them
- how he served as a tail gunner on 37 missions on a B-25
- how great the nurses were when they came to visit him and take his vitals

The ladies ate their lunches while paying courteous attention as Mel talked, and talked, and talked. I kept looking at my watch, wondering when he was going to stop. Finally, the director caught my eye and signaled to me by frowning and flicking her head toward the door. I knew what she meant. It was time to cut Mel off and take him home. I stood up and interrupted him.

"Well, this has really been a great opportunity for Mel to get to meet the hospice staff. I had better be getting Mel back home, as I'm sure he's probably getting very tired and would like to rest. Thanks so very much for permitting me to bring Mel over here."

I got behind Mel's wheelchair and proceeded to back him up a few feet and turn him around.

"Good-bye, Mel," they all said. Then several of them added, "Thanks for coming, Mel. It was nice to get to meet you. Good luck to you."

Minutes later I had Mel back in my car and was driving him home.

"That was nice, Joe. Thanks a lot for driving me over here. Now I know who all those hospice people are. You have a fine staff. But I didn't know they were all women."

"Most of the volunteers are women, too."

After I helped Mel into the house, I exchanged greetings with Catherine, told her briefly about Mel's meeting the hospice staff, and made my usual trip to the mailbox and left. I felt good about taking Mel to the hospice office. That was really something how he started talking and went on and on and on. What a gift of gab that guy has! I wondered what the hospice staff really thought about Mel monopolizing their meeting. But how Mel loved having them as an audience to listen to what amounted to being the story of his life.

Visit 5

A few weeks later I was back again inside the room addition chatting with Mel as he smoked cigarettes before his breakfast. The first thing I did was open four windows. It was still cold outside, with the temperature in the forties. Mel was dressed warmly, wearing a jacket and hat and had his blanket wrapped around his shoulders.

Catherine was leaving for another doctor's appointment.

"My hip is hurting especially bad today," she moaned. "I don't know what the problem is."

I sprang up from my chair.

"Can I back the car out of the garage for you?" I offered.

"Oh, I would like that very much," she said softly. "Here's the key."

Minutes later I had her Pontiac in the driveway by the back door. I was extra cautious in backing out. I didn't want any accidents.

"I left the motor running," I told her.

"Thanks, Joe, and God bless you. I'll be back in a couple of hours. Give Mel his breakfast as usual."

"Okay. Don't worry about a thing. I really like Mel, and he's continuing to get me good and broken in," I laughed.

"He keeps wanting to do something to earn his pay," Mel laughed. "I told him he can go out and clean up the garage and then dig around the bushes and start getting the house ready for painting," he laughed again.

"Mel, shame on you," Catherine chided. "Joe doesn't come here to work. He's just here to keep you company while I go on my errands."

"Well, he said he was looking for something to do. I was just trying to be helpful," Mel laughed.

I watched Catherine limp slowly out to her car.

"Your wife is a real sweetheart, Mel. Tell me

once again how that car accident happened."

"We were pulling out of this restaurant parking lot and turned left onto this highway. She was sitting by the left rear door, and I was sitting next to her. Our driver, a good friend of ours, pulled out right in front of this oncoming car, which struck us broadside right where Catherine was sitting. The impact just shattered her hip. She's had a number of surgeries to put everything back together. She'll probably have to have surgery again."

"You weren't hurt in the accident at all?"

"No. Catherine cushioned the impact for me. I didn't even get any bruises."

"Tell me again about your contracting cancer."

"I was diagnosed with lung cancer about six months ago."

"And, you smoked all your life—ever since you joined the service?"

"Yeah. I smoked all my life."

"Always smoked cigarettes?"

"Yeah. I tried to smoke cigars once, but I hated them. And I never could stand pipes."

"What brand of cigarettes did you smoke?"

"Just about any brand I could find. But my favorite brands were Lucky Strike and Camels."

"I notice that now you're smoking Marlboro's."

"Yeah."

"Well, let's see. If you started smoking at around age twenty, and you're eighty-one now, then you've smoked for sixty-one years!"

Mel laughed and went into a racking cough.

"Just think how much money you would have if you would have put into the bank the money you spent on cigarettes. You'd be a millionaire, wouldn't you?"

"Yeah, probably many times over," Mel grinned.

"Do you have any regrets about smoking for all those years?"

"No. I enjoyed every minute of it. I really like smoking. It's part of my life. I need a cigarette the first thing in the morning and the last thing at night. I always have, ever since I can remember."

A few minutes later I watched Mel eat his breakfast. He took only a few spoons of cereal and didn't touch his jam toast at all. Then he was back in his chair in the back room smoking another cigarette.

"How has that Norelco shaver been working?" I asked.

"It's on the blink again. I'm using the one in the bathroom with the plug-in cord."

"You mean the cordless actually worked good for a while after I put it back together?" I wanted to say, "after I fixed it," but if it wasn't working again, then I really hadn't fixed it.

"It worked for a couple of times after you fixed it, but then it quit on me again."

"It must have something wrong with the motor."

Just as I was about to have Mel tell me some more about his wartime experiences, Catherine's Pontiac stopped in the driveway by the back door. I watched her walk slowly into the room addition, and I held the door open for her.

"How was your doctor's visit?" I asked.

"It was okay. He wants to take another MRI and schedule me for some more surgery."

"Judging from the way you're walking, it must be awfully painful."

"Oh, it really is. It hurts terribly. I hardly get any sleep at night it hurts so bad."

"Mel has been telling me a lot of stories. But he didn't eat much breakfast."

"He didn't eat much breakfast? Shame on you, Mel. You know you're supposed to eat your breakfast."

"I wasn't hungry."

"That's not a good sign," Catherine whispered.

I went out to the mailbox and brought their mail in for them and was again on my way.

Visit 6

I again arrived at a few minutes before 11 o'clock. Catherine had called, asking me to sit with Mel while she went shopping with one of her daughters. After Catherine left with her daughter, I quickly settled into my routine with Mel. He was sitting in his rocker, and I was sitting on a chair facing him. I again opened several windows to rid the room of the smoke from his cigarettes. Although the temperature outside was in the low fifties, Mel still had on his jacket and hat and had a blanket wrapped around his shoulders.

"So how have you been, Mel?"

"I can't complain. It doesn't do any good if I complain, anyway," he laughed and then lapsed into a racking cough.

"I like your attitude, Mel—that you're going to whip your lung cancer. Are you feeling any better? Any worse?"

"Not any better and not any worse. Yeah, I'm going to whip this thing," he laughed again.

"Let's see, the doctor said you'd make it for a couple more months, didn't he?"

"Yeah."

"And, you're going to prove him wrong?"

Mel laughed again and went into another cough.

"How's your appetite been? Would you like to go in and have your breakfast?"

"All right, as soon as I finish this cigarette."

Minutes later I watched as Mel made his way slowly from his rocker and up the three steps into the kitchen.

"You seem to be walking okay, Mel. Maybe you're going to whip this thing after all."

I went out to my car and brought in my Thermos of hot tea and my peanut butter and honey sandwich. I went to the refrigerator and got out the little pitcher of milk that Catherine always left for his cereal. I sat down opposite Mel and launched into my sandwich and cup of tea. After only a couple spoons of cereal, Mel got up and poured himself a cup of coffee.

"Mel, you didn't touch your jam toast."

"I know. I just want my coffee, and I want to go back out to the porch and have another cigarette."

"Okay."

I watched Mel walk slowly to his rocker and sit down and light another cigarette.

"Would you mind if I opened a few more windows, Mel?"

"Nah. Open as many as you like."

"Mel, I don't believe I ever did ask you what kind of work you used to do before you retired."

"I worked at various jobs. Worked on a production line for a long time. Did some maintenance work. I retired when I turned sixty-five."

"Boy, you really led an interesting life, Mel. Your being raised in an orphanage. Your surviving those thirty-seven missions as a tail gunner on a B-25. Having your first wife die of cancer, and then being married to Catherine for thirty-one years. How did they treat you at the orphanage?"

"Real good. It was just like living at home."

"That must have really been tough, losing your first wife to cancer."

Mel went into another deep cough.

"Yeah. I don't think I ever told you, but our youngest daughter was killed in a car accident out west."

"Oh, my gosh! I'm sorry to hear that. How old was she?"

"Just in her early twenties. She was a real sweetheart."

I wanted to tell him that my wife and I had lost our 16-year-old son in a car accident 25 years ago. But I held back. After all, I wanted to hear Mel's story. He didn't need to hear mine.

"My first marriage—I was a real greenhorn. I didn't know anything about women."

Mel reached for his handkerchief to wipe away some tears.

"You really loved your first wife, didn't you?"

"Yeah. But I love Catherine, too."

He wiped some more tears away.

Pretty soon Catherine returned, and her daughter accompanied her into the house. Her daughter seemed shy around me but it was easy to tell she adored her mother. I went out to the mailbox and brought in their mail. Minutes later I was gone.

Several Weeks Later

Because of another commitment, I called Catherine at 8 o'clock in the morning to find out if she wanted me to sit with Mel today.

"No, Mel has taken a turn for the worse. He's getting very weak. He doesn't want to get out of bed, and he doesn't want to eat anything. I don't think I had better leave him."

I understood. After all, Mel was on hospice. He was dying. But wait a minute. Didn't Mel say the doctor told him he might make it for a few months more? What was happening? And hadn't Mel kept insisting he was going to whip his cancer and live for at least another year?

I went ahead and made plans to firm up my other commitment for the day.

A Week Later

I got a phone call this morning from the hospice office that Mel had died last evening. I was surprised; yet, somehow, I wasn't. When Catherine last called me, she knew Mel was dying. She loved him too much to leave him, to entrust him with anyone but herself.

A few days later I went to Mel's wake. Entering the parlor and walking slowly toward the casket, I looked around for Catherine to express my condolences. I spotted her talking with a priest I knew whom I hadn't seen for several years. I stood perhaps five feet or so away as they talked. Sensing motion in his peripheral vision, the priest turned to look in my direction and then turned back to look at Catherine. Then he did an abrupt double take and looked back at me, and we exchanged greetings. Then he went back to talking with Catherine, taking several notes, presumably facts about Mel for his funeral homily tomorrow. After expressing my condolences to Catherine, I knelt on the kneeler in front of the brown casket. Makeup gave the appearance that Mel was merely asleep. I studied his features. How handsome he appeared. His hair was combed neatly. He looked dapper in his pin-stripe navy blue suit with matching tie. A rosary with clear crystal beads was entwined in his fingers. Pictures of Catherine, of his children, and of her children were in the casket for viewers to see.

I mentally prayed something like this: Goodbye, Mel. Thanks for breaking me in. Thanks for telling me about the orphanage, about World War II, about some of your thirty-seven missions as a tail gunner on a B-25, about that 38th mission that you didn't go on, when your plane was shot down. Thanks for letting me open the windows while you smoked. Dear God, please grant Mel a high place in heaven. He did a good job here on earth. But, remember to open the windows for him. His smoke gets pretty thick.

I wiped at my tears as I left the funeral home. Yes, Mel did break me in. He broke me in real good. The following was printed on the back of Mel's "holy card" distributed at his wake:

I am home in heaven, dear ones;
Oh, so happy and so bright!
There is perfect joy and beauty
In this everlasting light.
All the pain and grief is over,
Every restless tossing passed;
I am now at peace forever,
Safely home in heaven at last.
There is work still waiting for you,
So you must not idly stand;
Do it now, while life remaineth-
You shall rest in God's own land.
When that work is all completed,
He will gently call you Home;
Oh, the rapture of that meeting,
Oh, the joy to see you come!

Copyright: Fratelli-Bonella

The front of the card shows a cemetery; a cross and plaque in the foreground states "In Memoriam"; an eagle holds an American flag; a Bible is on the ground in front of the plaque. The face of Jesus hovers in the upper right above and behind a willow tree.

The next day I attended Mel's funeral mass. I remembered from my hospice training that volunteers weren't expected to go to wakes and funerals. But I wanted to. I really grew to like Mel. I took a pew in the middle of the church and watched Catherine and her children and Mel's children and their spouses accompany the casket down the main aisle. Catherine didn't seem to be limping as much as usual. Had her pain subsided? Or was she stuffing her pain to make a good appearance?

After the service I wanted to leave right away but I couldn't. The funeral procession had the church parking lot exit blocked. I had to wait until the hearse and the entire funeral procession left the lot. I stood in front of the church and chatted with a woman who's car was also blocked. She told me she had been a friend of Mel and Catherine for a long time and had really liked Mel.

Several Weeks Later

I received a thank-you card from Catherine, which read:

Dear Joe,

You had a Lot of Love to give,—and you gave it to Mel! It was <u>so</u> wonderful that you could come— and be "HIS PAL"—we were very grateful!!

Mel was a Loving Husband—his greatest 'joy' was to brag about Our Large Family!

We were all happy he gypped cancer out of 2

more (predicted) months of suffering.

He loved—when you took him to visit 'hospice'—you Blessed us with "your presence"!

Thank you very much,
Catherine
My best to your good wife!

The printed message on the card read:
> Your kindness and sympathy
> in our recent sorrow
> will always be remembered
> with deep gratitude

Included with the thank-you card were two holy cards: one with Joseph holding the child Jesus, and one with Jesus in the Garden of Gethsemani, looking up at a ray of light and a chalice. The back of each card bore the same "I am home in heaven" poem.

Gladys

Ah, Gladys! I can't say enough about Gladys. She was my second hospice patient. I went to visit her for the first time after leaving the funeral for Mel, my first patient, who "broke me in."

Little did I realize on that first visit that I would be visiting Gladys once or twice a week for almost four years. I quickly found Gladys and her husband, Joe, her primary caregiver, to be so unusual that I wrote a book about them: *Gladys: Love Conquers Alzheimer's* (Infinity Publishing, 2002, 820 pages). Following are excerpts from the book:

April 27, 1999, Tuesday

Alzheimer's was ricocheting around the corners of my brain like a billiard ball searching for a pocket. What in the hell was this lethal disease that pummels the neurons of a healthy brain into chop suey, leaving its victims a hopeless vegetable? I was about to get a first-hand glimpse of its awful devastation....

(I found the house and was welcomed inside by a nurse's aide, who was waiting for me to arrive so she could leave.)

"So this is Gladys," I said. "Boy, she seems to be pretty bad off, doesn't she?"

"Yes, she has Alzheimer's real bad," she said, stretching out the word "bad" . . .

"She apparently can't communicate at all?"

"No. Well, every now and then she responds a bit. A little while ago I spoke to her and she seemed to answer me..."

I walked around to the right side of the bed and looked at the patient.

"Hello, Gladys," I said softly, smiling.

She looked at me momentarily, and then her vision left my face and drifted aimlessly about the room. She was making a guttural noise, alternating with a high-pitched undertone of syllables that only slightly sounded like words. Her bare arms and hands were in a constant slow motion, resembling a symphony maestro directing an adagio movement. She obviously didn't know if I were there or not. I spoke to her several times again and received the same response: nothing.

I went back to Gladys and tried speaking to her again, once again getting no response.

Minutes later I watched her (the nurse's aide) walk out to her minivan ...Then she was gone. That was it. I was on my own. It was going to be just Alzheimer's and me. Gladys was now my total responsibility. The only Alzheimer's patients I had ever seen before were on TV. I quickly reviewed my instructions: I shouldn't have to do anything for Gladys other than perhaps offer that juice (which had been left for her by her husband).

Gee, this ought to be easy. I began to pace slowly about the living room and kitchen, alternately glancing around me, at Gladys, and at the décor, ignoring the TV. I walked up to Gladys again.

"Hi, Gladys," I smiled. She began looking at me with intense interest, almost as though she were trying to figure out who I was.

"My name is Joe. I'm here to keep you company for a while. What can I do for you?" I smiled again. She continued to look intensely at me, still apparently trying to figure out who I was. She looked away and resumed making guttural sounds and soft-pitched noises that sounded something like singing softly to herself. Her head turned slowly back and forth, and she seemed to be looking at nothing in particular. Her fingers were busy playing with a pillow on her chest. I once again spoke to her, striving to communicate. I again got no response.

"So you've got Alzheimer's, eh, Gladys? What a tragedy! You look so young to have had your mind all but destroyed. Alzheimer's! Wow! I had no idea it left a person this bad off!" . . .

She was rather young looking. I would never have guessed her to be 70. Maybe 60, perhaps. Her rather small mouth was open most of the time. I didn't see any sign of her having teeth, and wondered if she had her own teeth, partials, full plates, or no teeth at all. Her lips were thin and not sensual. Her nose was thin and slightly aquiline. She had small and narrowly spaced gray-blue eyes. Her hair, straight and cut to about her shoulders, was brown with only a wisp or two of gray. A blanket, or perhaps it was an afghan, was covering her to just below her chin, revealing the top of what I figured must be a nightgown. Judging from where her toes pushed up the blanket, she seemed to be quite tall. I wondered if she were taller than I....

"Oh, my God!"

Her head and shoulders had slipped off her

43

pillow, coming to rest against the guardrail on the right side of her bed. Obviously she could not of her own power return herself to the pillow. I got on her left side and gripped under her neck with my right hand and her left shoulder with my left hand and tugged her back to the center of the bed. Boy, she's heavy! I wondered how much she weighed. Her neck felt stiff, and she seemed to watch me suspiciously as I pulled at her.

"It's okay, Gladys. I just put you back the way you were." She continued to study me intently, then resumed making her noises, looking about, waving her arms, and fingering her pillow. Then I remembered that I was supposed to give her a drink.

I studied the bed and figured that since it was a hospital bed, it must have one of those remote controls for elevating the head and feet. I readily spotted the control and pressed the "raise head" button and watched her upper body tip up to about 45 degrees. I went to the kitchen table to get the glass of juice and returned. Uh-oh. I'm going to need something to catch any spillage. I picked up one of about a dozen rolled-up towels on a small bedside table and tucked it under her chin and brought the glass to her closed mouth.

"Here's some nice juice for you, Gladys. Open your mouth for me."

She seemed to respond when the rim of the glass touched her lips. I slowly tipped the glass forward, letting a trickle of juice enter her mouth. I heard her swallow with a subdued noise that sounded like, "gunk." Success! Within a minute or so, the glass was empty. She swallowed it all nicely. And there had been no spillage.

"Good job, Gladys. You made that little job real easy for me." At least her Alzheimer's hadn't robbed her of her swallowing....

I went back to check on Gladys. Resting nearly horizontal, she looked very comfortable. She was still doing her thing. I stopped to speak to her, and her right hand pointed to the ceiling. I looked up and saw nothing but white. She seemed to be talking to something on the ceiling. I wondered what she was seeing. She was totally oblivious of me.

What do you see, Gladys?"

She continued to ignore me, apparently still speaking to the ceiling. I looked up again and felt some goose bumps forming on the back of my neck. Could she really be seeing something up there? An Alzheimer's vision? Then her arm lowered and her head once again began to turn back and forth, and she resumed fingering her pillow....

(At about 3 o'clock Joe, her husband, came home.)

"Hi. I'm Joe Schrantz, the hospice volunteer. You must be Joe, Gladys's husband," I smiled, looking into the gray-blue eyes of a white-haired man of about my height and build.

"Hi, Joe. Yes, that's me. How did everything go? Did you have any problems?"

"No. I gave her the juice that was on the kitchen table, and she drank it just fine." I felt immediately drawn to this man. He seemed to exude a warmth, like the sun in a clear sky on a cold day. I followed him to Gladys's bedside.

"Hi, babe. Everybody at the Club said to say

hello." He smiled lovingly down at his wife, who showed no awareness of his presence.

I watched slightly embarrassed as he leaned over and kissed Gladys on her open mouth.... "They all said to say hello, and they all said to tell you how much they miss seeing you," he said, kissing her on the mouth several more times. Gladys seemed to study him intently with her eyes while making no sign of recognition or indication that she had just been kissed half a dozen or more times. Another Alzheimer's trick: not to know when you've been kissed! . . .

"How long has she been like this?" I asked.

"Oh, she's had Alzheimer's now for about four years. But she's had it real bad for, let me see, maybe six months or so. She first contracted Alzheimer's when we were in Hawaii."

"Has the doctor estimated her life expectancy?" I asked hesitantly, feeling almost as though I were prying into his personal affairs.

"Anywhere from a month to a year or more." He paused and seemed to take in a deep breath. "I just hope I can keep her alive until May twenty-seventh of next year. That will be our fiftieth wedding anniversary." He glanced again at the catheter bag. "I better empty that." He bent down and drained the bag into a round, yellow plastic container. "Excuse me while I go empty this," he said, carrying the container to the bathroom.

I glanced at Gladys as I heard the toilet flush. She was again doing her Alzheimer's thing: moving her arms about, fingering the pillow, turning her head from side to side, mumbling and making a humming noise.

"Obviously she has a catheter," I said when he returned." Does she wear diapers?" I again felt as though I were intruding.

"Oh, yes. She can't get up to use the bathroom. It's about time for me to be changing her. I'll do that right after you leave," he said, stooping to place the plastic container on the floor beneath the bed....

"I was told by the hospice social worker that Gladys is seventy. Is that right?"

"Yes. And I'm seventy-five."

"You're seventy-five? Five years older? You sure don't look it." He smiled at the compliment as I studied his face again just to make sure that I really believed he didn't look his age....

"Can you come again next Tuesday?"

"I sure can." . . .

As I went out the front door, I told myself that I liked his warm handshake. I fact, I liked him, and I liked Gladys. But I hated this Alzheimer's! What a deadly beast! ...Driving home I felt good. I hadn't done hardly anything for Gladys, but my being there had permitted her husband to get out of the Alzheimer's shadow for a few hours. I wondered if his Tuesday Senior Club meeting was his only outing.

I began thinking about Alzheimer's. What a catastrophic disease! Poor Gladys. She's just out of it. Almost totally noncognitive. Practically a vegetable. How in the world did she contract Alzheimer's? Was it something she ate? Something she didn't eat? Something she drank? Something she didn't drink? Something she did? Something she didn't do? . . .

Easing my car into my driveway, a barrage of other questions exploded in my brain. Who is Gladys? What did she used to be like before her Alzheimer's? Had she been pretty? Who *is* her husband? What is compelling him to keep her alive until their fiftieth wedding anniversary? I did a hasty mental calculation. That's thirteen months from now! Why doesn't he farm her out to a nursing home? Then I remembered that he's five years older than his wife. Would Gladys outlive him? If so, who would care for her?

Somewhere off in the recesses of my brain I began to sense that I was being called on by fate to witness the final act of a great love story. Or, was it a love triangle? Joe, Gladys, and the satanic Alzheimer's.

The Weeks Go By

The weeks went by, and I continued to sit with Gladys on Tuesdays so her husband could attend his Club meetings for some much needed socializing. When I asked Joe for permission to write a story about him and Gladys, he didn't hesitate and said I could ask him anything I wanted. I began to come over to his house for a few days each week to interview him. The more interviews I did, the more I became fascinated with this story. I was simply amazed: Gladys, totally incapacitated, flat on her back, her mind destroyed by Alzheimer's, her husband her primary caregiver, she being the center of his life. His love for her blew me away. In July of 1999, because Gladys was doing so well, thanks mainly to her husband's loving care, she was removed from hospice and put on home health.

May 27, 2000, Saturday

As I prepared to leave my house for Joe's, I was excited. Today was May 27, Joe's and Gladys's 50th wedding anniversary! She had made it! Just 14 months ago Gladys left the hospital and entered a hospice program. Her physician had given up on her plugged-bowel condition and told Joe that she likely would be dead within a week. Gladys had defied the odds!

Joe had told me so many times, "If I can just keep her alive until our 50th wedding anniversary!" And here it was!

It was exactly 10 o'clock as I turned into Joe's driveway. Several cars were there . . .

"Hi, Joe. Happy 50th anniversary! Here's a card for you and a little gift," I beamed.

"Thanks. But you shouldn't have done it," he said, holding open the door for me.

"Oh, yes I should. This is a very important date. I think I'm more excited than you are." . . .

Entering the living room, there was Cathy (Joe's daughter) bending over her mother.

"Hi, Cathy. Hey, you're pinning on a corsage. That's neat. It's really pretty. What kind of flowers are they?" I asked, admiring two white flowers and a red one.

"I bought it at the Jewel Friday morning," Joe said.

"It's really pretty," I said.

"It isn't the corsage that I had wanted to buy.

Some lady picked out the one I wanted. This was my second choice."

"Doesn't she look pretty though! She's all ready for her big anniversary! Hey, she has on earrings. And, wait a minute! She has on a dress!" I was used to seeing her wearing a shift.

"Yes, she has on a dress. Cathy picked it out for her and put it on her."

I couldn't help but admire the dress. It had a lot of little black crescent-shaped designs on a white background. Only the top part of the dress showed above the blue angel afghan....

"And just look at those flowers!" I said, admiring a bouquet of salmon-colored roses in a vase on the small table on the left side of Gladys's bed. "Did you get her those, Joe?"

"No. They were sent by Sharon—that's Rich's wife. They're Korean roses!"

"Korean roses?"

"Yes. Korean roses are more delicate than our roses. Roses were always Gladys's favorite. That's why you see so many roses around here." . . .

After I finished taking pictures of Joe and Gladys, he asked me, "Do you think I should put a necklace on her?"

"Sure, by all means. This is a festive occasion. Yes, put a necklace on her."

Joe went to his bedroom and returned quickly with a pearl necklace and attached it around Gladys's neck.

"There, babe. Now you look like you're all ready for our anniversary. Don't you sweetheart? Huh? Don't you?" He bent over and kissed the upper lip of her open mouth. Gladys gave no visible sign that she was aware of either being kissed or of it being her 50th wedding anniversary....

"Here comes someone, Joe. Maybe it's Father Jim." I looked at my watch. It was 10:25. Joe sure called it right! He said Father Jim usually arrived at between 10 and 10:30. I went into the kitchen to meet Father Jim.

"Father, this is Joe Schrantz. He's been sitting with Gladys while I go to my Tuesday Senior Club meetings." . . .

Father Jim, bearing a little black bag, and Joe headed for Gladys, and I followed.

"Father Jim, would you mind if I took some pictures while you are with Gladys?"

"No, I wouldn't mind. That would be all right."

Father Jim put a stole around his neck and took out some holy oil and set about praying over Gladys. I picked up my camera and flash attachment and got in position and started taking pictures. I was wishing that I had my tape recorder with me to catch his ministrations. I remember that one of his prayers went something like this: "By the authority vested in me as a priest, I forgive you of all your sins, and by the authority vested in me by the Pope, I give you a plenary indulgence, meaning that you are freed from having to spend any time in purgatory." . . .

I went back into the living room and began to talk to Gladys... "Are you enjoying your fiftieth anniversary, Gladys?" She was mumbling/humming and looking straight ahead with her mouth open. "Just think, Gladys, now you have all your sins forgiven and a plenary indulgence to boot. Your soul is lily-white clean! If you die today, you'll go straight to heaven—nonstop. Wait a minute. What do I mean, if you die today you'll go straight to heaven? Because of your Alzheimer's, you can't possibly commit another sin, so that means that no matter when you die, you're going straight to heaven! Hey, that's neat, Gladys! The only thing keeping you from heaven is death itself."

The Summer of 2002

The weeks continued to whiz by, and pretty soon it was the summer of 2002. Gladys's health suddenly deteriorated. She simultaneously contracted pneumonia, a bladder infection, and a toxic reaction to one of her medications. She was put in the hospital. About a week later, she was sent back home and once again put on hospice. Several months later, because she once again was doing so well, she was again removed from hospice and put on home health. She had whipped the hospice odds a second time! Occasionally a hospice patient will show improvement and be removed from hospice. But how many beat the odds twice? Gladys did!

January 7, 2003

I continued sitting with Gladys on Tuesdays so Joe could attend his Club meetings. Things seemed to be going well, that is, until January 7, 2003, a Tuesday. My wife, Dorothy, had fallen in church on January 4, and broken her pelvis. She was hospitalized two evenings and was home on January 6. I asked her if she would be all right tomorrow while I sat with Gladys. She said I had to remain home and take care of her. I called Joe to tell him.

Early the next evening Joe called to tell me that Gladys had died. I was flabbergasted! How could that be? The last time I sat with her, she was fine, that is, she was her usual self! Joe told me about her dying:

"I had to miss my Club meeting and was staying home with Gladys. Early in the afternoon the hospice nurse came to check Gladys's vitals. Everything checked okay: her blood pressure, pulse, and respiration, and the nurse was sitting down in the living room filling out her paperwork when suddenly the inner front door opened—all the way, and the nurse said, 'Joe, your front door just opened. I think you have spooks.'"

Joe said he had been sitting at the kitchen table reading and got up and went to close the door. Minutes later the nurse left. About a half hour later, while Joe was still sitting at the kitchen table, he saw the living room inner front door open wide again. Joe said he went and closed it again.

"No way could that front door have opened by itself," Joe told me. "You know yourself how tightly that door closes. It's not about to open by itself."

Then, Joe said about half an hour later, as he was sitting in the living room chair where the nurse had been sitting, "Gladys spoke, saying, 'He's here.' I replied, 'Oh, he's here, is he?' And Gladys said, 'Uh-huh.' Then, a few minutes later,

Gladys starting breathing irregularly and suddenly took a deep breath, and passed away."

Having sat with Gladys for so many times, I can attest that there's no way she could speak. No way! Not a chance! Her brain was too riddled with Alzheimer's! But just before she died, she spoke!

"It was an angel coming to get her," Joe explained.

Then I recalled that Joe had countless angel figurines on various shelves around the living room, literally surrounding Gladys's hospital bed.

I pondered my not being with Gladys on the Tuesday she died. Oh, no! Could it be? Had heavenly forces caused my wife to fall in church Saturday just so I would have to stay home to look after her so I wouldn't be sitting with Gladys, so her husband could be with her on the day she was appointed to die? It was an intriguing question. When Dorothy fell, she was carrying a votive candle from the sacristy and fell down some altar steps, breaking her pelvis. She was to have placed the candle under the St. Anthony statue in church and lighted it, petitioning St. Anthony to help one of our grandsons. Could St. Anthony have been behind the plot: making Dorothy fall, just to keep me home with her to ensure that Gladys's husband would be with her when she died?

On Friday Gladys's wake and funeral were held, just as Joe had planned it several years earlier. She looked beautiful in her dress, earrings, and necklace. Her family was there. Countless friends from the Seniors Club came to pay their respects.

Several Weeks Later

Several weeks later I was visiting Joe, and he said, "There's Gladys."

I said, "What?" I looked around, expecting to see Gladys.

"Right there," Joe pointed to a small box on the little table that had rested alongside Gladys's hospital bed for over five years. "Her ashes."

Then I remembered. Joe had told me that Gladys was to be cremated.

"Can I pick it up?"

"Sure."

I lifted the box. It wasn't heavy, nor was it light. This was Gladys? I could feel myself getting choked up. This was the same Gladys I had sat with for so many Tuesdays, giving her water, juice, feeding her lunch, exercising her fingers, gently moving her arms about, rubbing her feet, talking to her.

I put the box down.

When I got home, I studied the remembrance holy card I had picked up at Gladys's wake and funeral. One side of the card had a painting of a cross and lighted candle, with five red roses and two yellow roses between the cross and candle, and a vine climbing the cross, with the word "Pax" next to the cross. These words were below the roses, "Like a Candle our life is consumed before the Face of Christ."

The other side of the card said:

In Loving Memory of
Gladys E. Kujawa
June 16, 1928 – Jan. 7, 2003
Services held at
Humes Funeral Home
Jan. 10, 2003   8:00 p.m.
Officiating
Deacon Dino Franch
Interment
Private

Gone is the soul that we have loved
And mother is at rest—
Her work is done; she sleeps in peace
Among the Master's blest.
Her work is finished on the earth
And her rewards are won
Nor should we weep or shed a tear
Because her work is done;
But rather we should face the world
As mothers always do
With eyes upturned to face the light
Of each kind day anew.

Bill

The hospice office phoned and asked me to contact Bill and visit him. The patient has colon cancer; a visit might free up his wife, enabling her to get out of the house. Bill tends to be irascible and might give me a hard time. I was encouraged to try to break through his irritability if I possibly could.

The next morning, with a bit of hesitancy, I phoned Bill. He said he had been asleep and was not a bit pleased that I had awakened him. He said he normally sleeps until noon because of his being up all night with diarrhea. I told him I was a hospice volunteer and had been assigned to contact him.

"If I could visit with you, perhaps I could bring you a bit of cheer, or maybe you could cheer me up," I laughed.

"Right now, all I want is my nurse. I don't want any hospice volunteers coming around."

I told him I would call back in the afternoon, but he told me not to call, that he had too many things to do.

I informed the hospice office that Bill just plain did not want me to visit him. The hospice office understood; it would find another patient for me.

I wondered about Bill. What did he look like? Why was he so angry? Then I thought, wait a minute, if I had colon cancer and had been up all night with diarrhea, wouldn't I be angry, too?

Todd

The hospice office phoned to give me another patient: Todd, 82, lung cancer, a resident of a nursing home. I called the nursing home and was told that visiting hours were from 8 to 8. I asked for and received directions to the place, because I wasn't familiar with the area.

Visit 1

I left home at 6:30 in the evening to visit Todd. I made a couple of wrong turns and for about 15 minutes was hopelessly lost. Somehow I got my bearings and finally found the place. I was not anxious to go in; I've never felt comfortable in a nursing home.

After signing in, I asked the young lady attendant if I could use a bathroom. She pointed to a key on a counter behind her. I picked up the key, attached to a stick about a foot long, and found the bathroom. After replacing the key, I set out to find Todd's room.

I headed down a long corridor with glistening floor tiles and smiled self-consciously at several elderly ladies sitting in wheelchairs. I turned right, into another long corridor, smiling at more ladies and a few men in wheelchairs, and then made another right, smiling again at patients in wheelchairs, and came to room 180.

The door was closed. A note attached to the door with a red thumbtack stated that Todd did not want to go to the dining room and needed assistance going to the bathroom. I opened the door and entered. A man, undoubtedly Todd, was sitting up in bed asleep, his head resting back on a pillow. He was wearing plastic-rimmed glasses. The TV was blaring loudly with a sitcom rerun.

I didn't want to wake him, so I sat down. Periodically his head would lower, as though he were taking a deep breath, and then his head would rest back on his pillow, all the while his eyes remaining closed. He had oxygen tubes in his nose. His blanket was down to his crotch, revealing what appeared to be a diaper.

I looked about the room, a private room with bathroom, and tried to ignore the TV. What should I do? Wake him? Wait for him to awaken? Leave? I looked at my watch. It was 7:25. I decided to leave and come back perhaps the next day. I opened the door and closed it and headed back down the corridors, smiling once again at the patients in wheelchairs. I felt almost guilty. There I was walking along as healthy as could be, and there they sat, helpless, but still able to muster up a smile for a stranger.

Six Days Later, Visit 2

I signed in at 2:10 p.m. at the nursing home and strolled down the corridor, making two right turns to room 180, smiling at a dozen or so people in wheelchairs. Most of them smiled back warmly and offered greetings.

When I entered the room, Todd said, "I'll bet that's the priest."

Four visitors were occupying chairs near his bed. Something prompted me to inject a little humor into the situation at hand. I stopped in my tracks and gave the sign of blessing just as a priest might do to let them think for a moment that I was indeed "the priest." Then I abruptly smiled.

"I was just joking. I'm not the priest," I laughed. "I was just pretending. I'm really a hospice volunteer come to visit Todd." I introduced myself and sat down in an empty chair. They laughed in a way that told me they were surprised; for an instant, they had really thought I was a priest.

A man and woman got up and excused themselves, saying they had to be going. The two remaining people introduced themselves as Todd's nieces. Then an attendant entered the room pushing a wheelchair. The woman in the wheelchair introduced herself as Lillian, Todd's wife. She said she had gone to the rest room.

I quickly noticed that the women referred to Todd as Toddie. He was speaking, but with difficulty, using oxygen all the while. His wife said he has emphysema.

I managed to get a conversation going with Todd. He said that during World War II he had served as a gunner/engineer on a B-24 bomber. He spoke with difficulty, getting out of breath quickly. I offered him two pieces of individually wrapped hard peppermint candy, which he took. He removed the wrapper from one and put the candy in his mouth and seemed to enjoy it. I told him I would bring him some more on my next visit. His wife said Wednesday afternoon was a good day to visit, and I mentally set next Wednesday when I would return.

I told a joke, which Todd said he didn't think was very good, that I would have to come up with something better. I promised him a better joke next time.

With a twinkle in his eye, he said he wanted to tell a *dirty* joke. With his wife and two nieces present, I said, "No, Todd, not now, there are ladies present." I couldn't get myself to call him Toddie.

"I'm going to tell it anyway," he smiled.

"No," I pleaded.

"A man once fell in the mud," he said, and we all burst out laughing.

"I want to tell another *dirty* joke," he said quickly. "The same man got up and fell in the mud again." We all laughed again.

"I like your sense of humor, Todd," I said.

He asked me to guess his age. I already knew from the hospice office that he was 82, but I told him, "You look like you might be, let me see, maybe about sixty or so," I said, trying to keep a straight face.

Smiling, he waved his hand upward, indicating that I was much too low.

"Sixty-five?"

He waved his hand upward again.

"Seventy?"

Again he waved his hand upward.

"Seventy-five?"

He was enjoying this immensely. He waved his hand upward again.

"Eighty?"

He laughed and waved his hand upward again.

"Eighty-two?"

"Yeah. That's right. Eighty-two," he smiled.

"Eighty-two? You sure don't look it," I fibbed.

"I'll be eighty-three in another month or so."

I made small talk with Todd and his wife and nieces for a while longer and then excused myself. "Todd, I'll see you next Wednesday. And I'll bring you some more hard candy and some more jokes. And next time my jokes will be funnier," I laughed. "But please don't tell any more dirty jokes," I laughed again.

Before I left, Todd insisted I take along a sheet of paper containing the following free verse:

"I'll do roly-polys in the snow
when I'm 87.
Is it fun at 87?
I think I'll go wild when
I'm old and quite eccentric.
Yes, I'd like that!
I'll go singing in the rain,
(something I've always wanted to do)
with bright yellow galoshes on and a red hat.
When you're old, they just say,
'Poor old dear, she's not got long to go,'
and tap their heads.
So you see, I could do all the things
but couldn't do, because I was young.
Be like a little child at eighty-seven.
Jump in haystacks and pick flowers from
other people's gardens.

Do roly-polys in the snow.
I could have quite a bit of fun,
when I'm old."

(author unknown)

The Next Day

At midmorning the hospice office called to tell me Todd had died during the night. I couldn't believe it. I had just chatted with him last evening. He had all his faculties. I was supposed to visit him again next Wednesday.

Todd's obituary was in the morning's paper. Since I had other commitments, I didn't go to either his wake or to his funeral. Todd didn't make it to 87, and he didn't do roly-polys before he died. But he kept his sense of humor right up to the end. Wait a minute. Maybe his "dirty" jokes were roly-polys.

Dan

Visit 1

The hospice office called to assign me a new hospice patient. The thumbnail description: a man, 81, lung cancer, has two daughters, one who stays with him much of the time; his wife died five years ago.

Right after she hung up, I called the patient's residence and spoke with his daughter Therese. Her voice was pleasant and exuded a warmth. She consulted with her father and told me, "Sure, it's okay if you come over at eleven o'clock today."

This was, indeed, fast work for me. I don't usually set up an appointment with a hospice patient this quickly.

I arrived at the residence, a town house, a few minutes before 11, parking on the street. The building, red brick, was in the middle of a block. I walked up six or seven steps to a concrete stoop and rang the doorbell.

"Hi, my name is Joe Schrantz, and I'm a hospice volunteer. You must be Therese, with whom I spoke on the phone," I smiled.

"Yes. I'm Therese. Please come in."

She was attractive, had a trim figure, and I judged her to be about 50.

I showed her my hospice volunteer badge. "This makes me official," I laughed.

"My dad is in the kitchen with Peggy, his nurse. She's checking his vitals."

"I know a hospice nurse named Peggy. I wonder if this is the same nurse," I said.

I followed her through the living room into a small kitchen. The nurse and Dan were sitting at the kitchen table, and the nurse was using a stethoscope to listen to his heart. She looked up at us.

"Hi, Peggy," I smiled. "Nice to see you again."

"Hi, Joe. Nice to see you again, too," she replied.

"Dad, this is Joe Schrantz, the hospice volunteer."

I stepped up to him and reached out a hand.

"Don't bother to get up," I told him. We shook hands, and I thought his grip was a little soft. "Nice to meet you, Dan."

"Nice to meet you, too," he said. I thought his smile was a bit forced.

He spoke with some difficulty, as though he were in pain. He had thinning gray hair and nice features. His face looked a bit flushed. He had a reserve about him, as though he might be depressed. Well, wouldn't I be depressed, too, if I were 81 and on hospice with lung cancer?

"Sorry to interrupt you," his daughter said. "Come on, Joe, let's go wait in the living room until Peggy finishes with Dad."

I followed her into the living room, where she stretched out on her left side on a single bed along the north wall. I concluded that this must be where Dan slept. I took a seat in a stuffed chair nearby.

"Tell me about your dad," I smiled. I thought

the brown bedspread matched the color of her eyes.

"Dad was admitted to hospice only last week and was given a year or so to live. He parachuted behind enemy lines a day before D-Day in the invasion of Normandy in World War II."

"No kidding!" A year or so to live? People put on hospice were usually given less than six months. I wanted to question her on this, but thought it would be indiscreet.

"He was at a meeting in an abandoned schoolhouse when a German shell exploded, killing two of his comrades. The explosion hurled their bodies on top of him, and when the medics came, they tagged my dad as dead. But other than being knocked unconscious, he had only minor injuries. For this he received the Purple Heart."

She was interrupted by a phone call, which she said was from her son. She explained that she was very sad that day because their old chocolate lab was being put to sleep.

Ten minutes or so later Peggy the nurse came into the living room and sat down and chatted with us. Suddenly Therese jumped up.

"Oh, my God! I just remembered. I have to pick up my son."

Dan entered the living room after stopping at a bathroom, readily visible through an open door from the living room, and sat down in a recliner in front of a large TV set, which was turned on. Then the nurse left, as did his daughter.

For a few moments I tried to communicate with Dan from where I was sitting, but it wasn't working. He seemed to be a bit hard of hearing, and the TV was turned up rather loud. I got up from the chair and moved closer to Dan, sitting on the second to last step on a stairway leading upstairs.

My moving closer to him eliminated the obstacle of distance. Now I had to overcome the next obstacle: the loud TV. Dan seemed to be wavering as to which to watch: the TV or me. The TV was winning. Maybe if I could get him to start talking—

"Tell me a little bit about yourself, Dan. Your daughter told me that you parachuted behind enemy lines the day before D-Day in Normandy."

"Yeah, that's right." He looked at me momentarily and then stared back at the TV. I was losing to the TV.

"That plane that you jumped from must have been flying pretty low to prevent the Germans from seeing you and shooting you as you came down."

"The plane was flying at only a hundred and fifty feet above the ground."

"What was it, a C-47?"

"Yeah."

"Wow! You must have hit the ground only moments after your chute opened."

"That's right."

I was winning.

"You say you parachuted behind enemy lines the day before D-Day. What was your mission?"

"Our mission was to wipe out a German bastion and clear out a causeway."

"A causeway?"

"Let me turn off the TV," he said, aiming his remote at the screen. The TV went silent and dark. I had won!

"It was a rather narrow strip of land where the Germans were located in a heavy concentration."

"Did you accomplish your mission?"

"Yes. The Germans fled. They thought they were grossly outnumbered."

"Then, what did your group do the next day, D-Day?"

"We were the parachute infantry. We spearheaded through enemy lines, leading the D-Day invasion force."

"Boy! Is that ever exciting! And, to think you actually survived!"

"Some months later our outfit jumped into Holland and were caught in the Bastogne Battle of the Bulge."

"You were in the Battle of the Bulge? I remember from news reports during World War II that that was one fierce battle, that the Germans had our forces trapped there for some time."

"Yeah."

"You must have been one tough soldier to survive D-Day and the Battle of the Bulge!"

Dan smiled. "Yeah, I was pretty tough."

"What kind of weapons did you carry when you jumped from the plane?"

"I had a carbine, hand grenades, and a lot of survival equipment. When I jumped, my backpack weighed a hundred and sixty pounds."

"Wow! And how big were you at the time?"

"I was five-eight and weighed about a hundred and forty-five."

"Your backpack was heavier than you," I laughed.

"Yeah," he smiled.

I showed Dan my hospice badge.

"This proves I'm official," I laughed. I put the badge back in my pocket.

"I see that your town house faces the jogging trail. I used to ride my bike along here quite a bit. I would ride as far as Patterson. But one day just this side of Patterson, four black guys yelled at me from about half a block away, 'Hey, white boy. What you doing in this area? You better get the hell out of here.' So I did. I got out of there in a hurry. Thank God they didn't come after me."

"The blacks are too bossy. They're always going out of their way to insult white people."

We were really conversing now. Then the phone rang. It was on a small table near his chair, and he picked it up. He spoke into the phone for several seconds and then hung up.

"That was my nephew. He's coming over to fix the rearview mirror on my car."

"Do you still drive?"

"I don't like to drive anymore because of the morphine I take. It makes me real dopey."

"What kind of work did you do before you retired?" I asked.

"I worked for twenty-five years or so in a pottery business, making clay pots, preparing them and firing them, making thousands a day. I left the business after it began to decline. Then I went to work as a maintenance man for some apartments located near where a famous resort hotel used to be. I got to know the former owner of one of the professional football teams, who lived in the apartments, and got his autograph."

"Yeah? How about that! When did you learn you had lung cancer?" I asked hesitantly, fearing that Dan might think I was prying.

"Eight months ago I had a heart bypass operation. In the process of X raying me, they found some dark spots on my lungs and identified them as cancer. It was already in a pretty advanced stage. I have a cracked or broken rib from the cancer, or from the heart surgery, I don't know which. I'm in a lot of pain from it."

"A cracked or broken rib? Boy, there's supposed to be nothing more painful than an injury to a rib!"

"I can walk only a little ways before I get out of breath."

"Are you on oxygen?"

"I just use it when I feel short of breath."

"I used to work with a lady who told me her mother had whipped breast cancer by eating a lot of carrots. But, wait a minute. I always get the story mixed up. I'll give her a call and get the story straight and tell it to you on my next visit."

"I've been given a couple of books about how to defeat cancer. One of them is over there on that little table by the door." Dan reached to his left and picked up a flyer from a table. "Here's a page from a tabloid newspaper containing an advertisement about a book on how to defeat cancer by eating a certain type of diet. I think the diet contains a lot of linseed oil. But how could linseed oil do any good? I think linseed oil is used in paint."

Minutes later the nephew walked in the front door. He was a big man, probably about 55. Dan got up from his chair and seemed to hint that my visit was over.

"Would you like for me to leave now?" I asked.

"Yes. That would be nice. We have to go out to my car."

"Okay. Let's see, about my next visit. I'm going to be tied up until Saturday. How about if I give you a call?"

"Okay, that would be nice."

On the way out to my car I noticed a big Chrysler parked in front of my car. It must belong to his nephew.

When I got home I looked at the advertisement for the book: "How to Fight Cancer and Win," William L. Fischer, copyright 1999, Agora Smith, Inc. Agora Health Books, Dept. 1810, P.O. Box 977, Frederick, MD 21705-9938. $19.95 plus $4.00 for shipping. Maybe I would send for it.

Visit 2

I arrived at Dan's town house at 2 o'clock as scheduled. Dan met me at the front door and invited me in. He went right to his recliner in front of his big TV set, and I, with his permission, brought a chair from the kitchen and placed it near to him. He then turned off the TV, for which I was glad.

"Did you find out about that carrot story?" he

asked right away. I was surprised he had remembered.

"Yes, I did. I called my friend, with whom I used to work, and had her tell me the story again. Some years ago, her mother was diagnosed with breast cancer. She went through the usual mastectomy, had the breast removed, and the lymph glands under her arm. And right away someone talked her into drinking a lot of carrot juice. She drank from six to eight huge glasses of carrot juice a day for five or six months, and her skin actually started turning orange. My friend said she and her sister bought a lot of organic carrots and made juice out of them in a blender."

"Is that the only kind of food she had—carrot juice?"

"No. My friend said she ate other foods besides, but continued with the big glasses of carrot juice every day. Anyway, her cancer never recurred. Of course, maybe the cancer would not have come back whether or not she had the carrot juice. Who knows? But my friend said her mother lived for twenty to twenty-five years after that.

"And she told me another story, about a man who had leukemia. He started drinking carrot juice and the leukemia went away. She said he drank a lot of it, something like the amount that her mother drank. And his leukemia was still in remission five years later.

"But here's an exciting part of my phone call to my friend to get that carrot story straightened out. I was telling her about you, how you had parachuted with the 101st Airborne Division behind enemy lines the day before D-Day. And, of all things, you could have knocked me over, but she said *her* husband was also with the 101st Airborne and parachuted into Normandy *on* D-Day."

"Is that right? What is his name?"

"Her husband's name is Mike Smith. He's a real big guy."

"Mike Smith? No, I never knew a guy in our division by that name. But I remember we had some real big guys in our outfit."

"Well, maybe one of those big guys was her husband," I smiled. "Oh, by the way, my friend told me the 101st Airborne Division is mentioned in the 'Private Ryan' movie."

"Yeah. Isn't that something. Oh, a couple of days after you were here, I went to the health food store and bought a quart of carrot juice."

"How much did you drink?"

"Just a glass a day."

"My friend's mother drank six to eight big glasses a day."

"That's too much," Dan said, shaking his head. "One glass a day ought to be sufficient."

We started talking about health food, and Dan pointed out to me that on page 55 of his cancer-prevention book it tells about a Japanese mushroom called maitake.

"It's supposed to have powerful anticancer properties."

Dan had me write down a description of the mushroom and asked me if I would take him to a nearby health food store so he could try to buy some. I was delighted he asked me to do something for him.

He walked out to my car with very little help from me. I gently held his arm walking down his porch steps. After a pleasant drive to the health food store, I found a parking place right near the door. We went inside, and Dan picked out another quart of carrot juice and a bottle of the maitake pills, which cost over $30. I bought some sunflower seeds, flax seed, and a quart of carrot juice. I didn't really want the juice, but bought it to impress Dan.

On the way back to his town house, I told him a little about my own family, how my wife and I have seven daughters but lost a son some years ago in a car accident when he was only 16. He expressed great sympathy for our loss. We arrived back at his town house at 3:30.

I went with him into his kitchen and watched him put his food away. I asked him about what I thought were hypodermic needles on his kitchen table.

"They're not needles. They're a new type of device to inject morphine pain medication into the mouth and swallow it. It will knock the pain out in ten to fifteen minutes. My damaged rib really causes me a lot of pain, especially when I'm in bed and try to turn over."

Something, probably his trim figure, prompted me to ask Dan if he played golf.

"I used to be an avid golfer and shot mostly in the eighties. I used to have a collection of about twenty-five putters, including one handmade in St. Andrew's, Scotland. I bought it at a resale shop for only two dollars. I found out later that that same putter sold at retail for a hundred and sixty-three dollars."

"No kidding!"

"I still have several sets of golf clubs."

"Do you still play?" I thought that was a dumb question. How could he play golf in his present condition?

"No."

"What was the best shot you ever made?"

"I remember it just like it was yesterday. It was a six iron on a par four. It was my second shot, and the ball went on the green and into the cup for an eagle."

"No kidding!"

I told Dan I eat a lot of grain, and he said he couldn't eat seeds because of his diverticulitis. I told him what I typically have for breakfast: two pieces of whole-grained wheat bread with honey and something healthy sprinkled on the honey, such as granola, sesame seeds, sunflower seeds, or soybeans, and an apple, a carrot, and four or five dried prunes. He was amazed.

"Do you eat the prunes for a laxative?"

"No, not really. I just like the taste of them, and they're supposed to be very good for you. I stay regular whether I eat the prunes or not."

"Speaking of being regular," he said, "recently I didn't have a BM for five days."

"Five days?"

"Yeah. I called the hospice nurse, and she came out and put a rubber glove on and inserted a finger into my rectum to break up the hardened material. That did the trick, because later I had my BM and then resumed my normal BM habits."

I noticed a nasty bruise on his upper left arm and asked him about it. He said it was caused by bumping the arm. I didn't push him for a deeper explanation.

The phone rang and it was Dan's grandson Zachary. They chatted for a few minutes until Dan cut him off, telling him a social worker was here. I didn't know I was a social worker!

"My family is very close to one another," he said.

I complimented Dan for his fervor and determination to whip his cancer. I compared his efforts to a game, but a game much more real and exciting than golf.

The phone rang, and it was the hospice chaplain. Dan said he would be arriving in about 15 minutes. I told him I would stay until he arrived. When his doorbell rang, I let him in and shook his hand. He recognized me from my hospice training.

Before leaving, I agreed to visit Dan again at 2 p.m. next Monday. But then he remembered that that was a holiday and suggested I skip a visit next week. I told him I'd call him, and left my name and number with him so he could call me whenever he liked.

Nine Days Later

I had called Dan over the weekend and we agreed I should visit him today. I stood on his front porch ringing his doorbell at 2 o'clock. I rang the bell three or four times but no one answered. I sat in my car for about five minutes and returned and rang the bell three or four more times. Again there was no answer.

What was the problem? Was Dan inside but unable to come to the door? Had he gone out? Had he died? I was genuinely concerned, as he had consented to my visit.

I went home and phoned him and left word on his tape recorder that I had been there at 2 o'clock but got no answer when I rang the doorbell. I then called his daughter Therese and expressed my concern to her. She apologized for her father, stating that her son Zachary was taking her father out for a ride, that apparently Dan had forgot his appointment with me. I told her I really enjoyed visiting and chatting with her dad and was hoping we could schedule another visit.

Two Days Later

Dan phoned and apologized for not being home when I went to his town house. We reset our visit for 2 o'clock Monday. I told him he needn't apologize, that if I were him, I would much rather have gone out with my grandson, too.

Visit 3

I arrived at 2 o'clock and was let in by a woman who identified herself as Millie, a hospice nurse. She told me to have a seat while she went back to the kitchen to finish checking Dan's vitals. I went to the kitchen and peeked in.

"Hi, Dan."

"Hi, Joe."

"I'll go sit in the living room and wait until Millie finishes with you," I smiled.

In the living room I looked out the front door and then paced around, glancing at wall pictures and various artifacts. Then I sat down and began to page through Dan's book on how to defeat cancer.

Millie made her exit at 2:20, and Dan invited me into the kitchen to chat.

"I brought you a little gift," I told him. "A loaf of whole-grained wheat bread I bought at the supermarket. I eat it regularly and keep mine in the freezer and eat two slices every morning with honey on them along with various things, such as soybeans, sesame seeds, sunflower seeds, or granola."

He wanted to pay me for the bread, but I objected.

"I haven't been breathing too well today and have been on oxygen most of the day," he apologized.

I offered to drive him back to the health food store, but he wasn't too sure he could make it due to his bad breathing. After chatting a while, during which time he didn't use his oxygen, he agreed to have me take him to the health food store. He walked out to my car readily, holding my arm only while walking down his front steps and while getting into my car.

At the health food store, he bought two cartons of carrot juice, and I bought one carton, along with some soybeans (garlic and onion flavored) and some organic raisins.

We returned to Dan's town house, and he again took my arm getting out of the car and going up his front steps. When we got to his kitchen, he was panting furiously. At his direction, I turned on his oxygen machine. After breathing in the oxygen for a few moments, his breathing returned to normal.

While we made small talk, he had several spells of deep coughing peculiar to lung cancer.

"My breathing's got worse the last few days," he apologized.

I suggested I leave so he could get some rest. He seemed very tired.

"Okay if I come back for another visit in a week?"

"That would probably be all right. But since I'm feeling so awful and my breathing's got so bad, maybe I better not make a commitment."

"That's okay, Dan. Tell you what. I'll give you a call on Monday at about noon to see if you feel up to a visit. If you're feeling okay, I'll come again at 2 o'clock. How'd that be?"

"Sounds good."

"Well, Dan, it's three-thirty, and I think I had better go so you can get some rest. I think I wore you out," I laughed.

As I drove home, I thought about Dan. He didn't seem to be in as good spirits as he was the last time I visited him. Maybe because of his increased difficulty in breathing. I said a silent prayer for him.

Six Days Later

Dan called me at about 5:30 p.m. "Joe, I don't think you better come for your visit on Monday. I have a doctor's appointment, and besides, the nurse will be coming over. Also, my breathing has got a lot worse. I'm taking oxygen all the time."

"I'm sorry to hear that you're doing so poorly, Dan. I hope you start feeling better. Say, have you tasted that whole wheat bread yet?"

"Which bread?"

"That loaf of bread I left for you."

"Oh, that. No, I haven't tried it yet."

"Well, when you do try it, you'll be in for a treat. It's really delicious."

Before hanging up, I told him, "Thanks for calling me, Dan. You really brightened my day. I'll plan on seeing you then on the following Monday, okay?"

"Okay."

"Good-bye, Dan."

"Good-bye."

After hanging up, I said another silent prayer for him.

Three Days Later

The hospice office called while my wife and I were out and left word on our tape recorder that Dan died Thursday evening. I was considerably shocked, because Dan and I had agreed to meet the following Monday.

I dialed the number of Dan's daughter

Therese. She was out and I found myself talking with her son Zachary.

"I'm the hospice volunteer who has been visiting with Dan, and I just wanted to express my sadness over his death. I really liked your grandfather."

"Yes, he was cool," Zachary said.

I asked him to tell me about Dan's death. He said something like the following: "I got to his town house at about seven-fifteen, and Grandpa was lying on the bed in the living room. My mother, her sister, and the rest of the grandchildren were all there. We were watching TV, and Grandpa seemed to be quite comfortable. I remember looking over at him at about seven-thirty and noticed that he seemed to take a deep breath. Then he died. He died a beautiful death."

I called the hospice office and expressed my thoughts about Dan's dying, telling her how I had grown to like him and to look forward to our meetings.

Three Days Later

I arrived at about 4 o'clock at the funeral home to attend Dan's wake. I went right up to the casket and knelt down to say a prayer. He looked distinguished, with suit and tie, and a rosary entwined about his fingers. My prayer went something like this: I'm so glad I got to know you, Dan. I just pray that you may have a high place in heaven. Thanks for telling me about a couple of your World War II adventures. What amazing adventures they were! And thanks for letting me drive you to the health food store.

Finishing my prayer, I went up to his daughter Therese. I hadn't seen her since my first visit with Dan. She was delighted to see me and called me by my first name. Minutes later she introduced me to her sister, remembering my name. I was impressed.

"Thank-you so very much for visiting Dad. A few days before he died he asked me for a slice of that whole wheat bread you brought him. He said, 'I just as well try it. What the heck.' After he ate a slice, he said he liked it a lot," Therese said.

"Hi, you must be Zachary," I said, walking up to him and holding out my hand. He was a really nice looking young man, several inches taller than I, with a crew cut, rimless glasses, and a look of deep self-assurance. His mother had referred to Zachary as "his grandfather's beer-drinking buddy."

Zachary told me another of his grandfather's war stories. "One time he was in a foxhole when a shell exploded nearby, burying him alive. Lucky for him, one of his comrades dug him out, saving his life."

As I chatted with Zachary, Therese's other children, Caleb and Sarah, came up and introduced themselves to me.

As I left the funeral home, I picked up a "holy card" announcing Dan's death. The picture showed the young Mary holding the child Jesus. The picture was painted by a famous Italian, whose name escapes me. But I read a story recently in St. Anthony magazine about the picture. The model for Mary was a girl of about 12, and the model for the child was her baby brother. The girl later was taken to the United States with her family, and became a nun. In her later years the nun went back to Italy to discover her roots. The back of the card read:

You are not forgotten, loved one
Nor will you ever be,
As long as life and memory last
We will remember thee.
We miss you now, our hearts are sore
As time goes by we'll miss you
more.
Your loving smile, your
gentle face,
No one can fill your vacant place.

As I drove home, I thought about Dan. What a nice man! How did he ever survive D-Day and the Battle of the Bulge? How blessed I was to get to meet him and spend a little time with him before he died. A conflict the next day prevented me from attending his funeral.

Eddie

At about 11:30 a.m. the hospice office called and asked if I would pick up a prescription and deliver it to the home of a new hospice patient, Eddie, 1020 S. Taylor, an apartment on the third floor on the west side of the street, and I am to ring the top bell. Eddie has lung cancer and lives with his sister, Patricia. I was given the apartment's phone number in case I had any problems. The prescription had just been phoned in to the pharmacy, and I was told to wait about an hour before leaving to pick it up. The patient's sister was told that I would arrive with the prescription between 1 and 2. Eddie's lung cancer has metastasized, meaning it has spread throughout his body.

I left my house at 12:45 for the pharmacy, mentally planning my route: to the pharmacy, south on Taylor to 1020, and return home along Jefferson. It would be a piece of cake. So I thought.

I found a convenient parking place at the pharmacy, showed my hospice volunteer badge, signed for the prescription, and was back in my car and heading for 1020 S. Taylor.

But I couldn't find 1020 S. Taylor. A strip mall at the southwest corner of Taylor and Jefferson had 1018, a Chinese carryout restaurant, and 1022, a print shop. I saw a three-story building just behind the strip mall and drove to it, but saw no name on the doorbells that resembled that of my patient, nor an apartment number like 3C, which was on the prescription. I went back to my notes and verified the address. I had become thoroughly frustrated. I just couldn't find 1020 S. Taylor!

I found a phone at a nearby gas station and called the number of Eddie's apartment. I told his sister where I was, that I could not find 1020 S. Taylor.

"You're looking for 1020 on the south side of Haven? We live on the south side of Randport!"

Then it hit me. When the hospice office told me 1020 S. Taylor, she undoubtedly told me Randport, but my brain probably tuned her out and immediately pegged the address in Haven. Oh, boy! Did I feel stupid! I had wasted 45 minutes looking for an address in the wrong town!

I headed up Taylor and 10 minutes later parked behind the three-story apartment building on the south side of Randport with the address of 1020 S. Taylor. I rang the top doorbell, 3C, and a buzzer opened the door. I hiked up three floors and Patricia let me in. At last, I had found it!

She was a pleasant-looking, Mediterranean-appearing woman of about my age. I showed her my hospice badge and told her I had her prescription. She didn't know anything about the medicine, and I had to figure it out for her. It contained some "syringes" that resembled hypodermic needles, but which were actually little siphon pumps. I showed her how to work them. She had two small bottles of medication and was supposed to give Eddie a full syringe of one, and half a syringe of the other. A visiting nurse had written the names of two medicines on a piece of paper, but only one of the names of the two medicines matched.

To dispel any doubt, I called a nurse at the hospice, and she told me the one name was generic, and the other was a trade name. So, the correct medication had been delivered! I watched as Patricia siphoned out a full syringe to give to her brother. At first, he wouldn't take it, probably thinking it was a hypodermic needle. After I told her to reassure him it wasn't a needle, he opened his mouth, and she squeezed in the contents of the syringe. Then she gave him half a syringe of the second medicine. I checked the medication: one was a narcotic for pain, the other, a sedative for anxiety.

Eddie was thin, with balding, gray hair. He was lying on his back on a hospital bed, clad only in diapers. The living room was very warm, and he obviously was warm. His sister said he had been sleeping off and on. I went over to look at him, and he appeared to be asleep. Or was he comatose? He had oxygen tubes leading into his nostrils. He coughed frequently, those terrible-sounding deep coughs peculiar to lung cancer.

I sat down and began to chat with Patricia about her brother. He had been in hospice for about a week; his lung cancer had disabled him only recently. Quite active prior to that, he had done a lot of walking. She said she and her brother had smoked almost all their lives, quitting only recently. Her brother had been a factory worker, retiring when he turned 62. He was now 70, and she, 72.

I was curious about why they both looked Mediterranean but had an Irish-sounding name.

She explained that their father had emigrated from a Mediterranean country, and when people in the United States had difficulty spelling his name, he decided to change it to something simple, not realizing that he had inadvertently chosen an Irish name.

She said it is very difficult caring for her brother, that just last night he had wandered around and had fallen, and she had one dickens of a time getting him up and back into bed. She didn't know how she picked him up, lifting all that "dead weight."

I asked her how long her brother was expected to live, and she quoted the nurse as saying he would likely die this week. I told her that if I could be of any help, to give me a call. I left my name and phone number.

The Next Day

The hospice office called to tell me Eddie had died during the night. Because of other commitments, I did not make it to his wake or to his funeral.

Tony

I was assigned another hospice patient: Tony, 84, lives with his son, Tony Jr., in a second-floor apartment across a street from a funeral home; colon cancer for two years, refuses radiation and chemotherapy and doesn't want to go to doctor or hospital; has one kidney, appetite good, very weak, sleeps most of the day, often constipated, unable to sit up, Catholic.

I pondered the information. I wasn't optimistic about visiting him, thinking that it could be very unpleasant.

I phoned his apartment and found myself speaking with his son. He said it would be all right to visit his father at 11 a.m. on Wednesday. I was told the apartment front door is never locked, to go in, and I would find his dad in the bedroom on the left.

Visit 1

At a few minutes before 11 o'clock, I entered the front door, calling Tony's name and announcing who I was.

"Come on in," a pleasant voice called out from the bedroom.

I entered through the living room. I could see the kitchen off to the right. I passed the open door to the bathroom on the left and the closed door to another bedroom on the right.

"Hi, Tony. My name is Joe Schrantz, and I'm a

hospice volunteer. Your son said it would be all right to visit you today. How are you?"

I was looking at a handsome man who didn't appear to be 84. He looked more like 64. He was lying on his back with his head on several pillows and covered up to his neck with a blanket. The head of his hospital bed was raised slightly. The bedroom was fairly small. A low dresser or table on the right held some pictures and medicine containers. A portable tray was over the foot of the bed, and a commode was on his left. A stuffed chair was in the left corner, and a high dresser was against the wall on my left. A horizontal row of windows was above and behind his bed, with the venetian blinds closed. I detected traces of the intestinal odor I feared would be present.

I went up to him and we shook hands. He had a warm handshake and a large hand. I couldn't get over how handsome this man was. And he looked so young. I was struck immediately by his pleasant voice. Only a salesman could have a voice like that. I quickly found out that he indeed had been a salesman all his life. He instructed me to bring in a chair from the living room and sit down. When I went to get the chair, I was impressed by the beauty of a family portrait on the wall behind the chair, showing a young couple with three small children. I figured, correctly, that this was an old picture of Tony and his wife with their young children. Tony was extremely handsome in the picture; his wife wore a fur coat, and little Tony Jr. wore a bow tie. How old was the picture? It had to be about 45 years old. I thought the apartment seemed very warm, and a glance at the temperature on the nearby wall thermostat told me I was right. It read 78.

I got him to talking about himself and found out the following:

- His wife, Kay, died 11 years ago at age 72 of what Tony described as a skin disease. Tony is to be buried alongside her.
- He has lived with his son five years in this apartment complex, the first two years in a downstairs apartment. He used to have an apartment above a store in another suburb.
- Three children in their fifties: Kay, the oldest; Wilma, next to oldest; and Tony Jr.
- Tony used to run a one-man business, selling medical products. His son has taken over the business.
- Tony said his father's family originated in a Mediterranean country.
- Tony was born in Oklahoma. He had three brothers and three sisters. Still living is an older sister and a younger sister.
- Tony is approximately 5-10.

Our small talk was interrupted by Tony Jr. entering the front door and coming into the bedroom. He was handsome, but he lacked the sophisticated handsomeness of his father. He said he just dropped in to meet me. After we exchanged pleasantries and he presumably checked me out and was satisfied with what he saw, he said he was leaving. After his father told me that Tony Jr. drives a sports car import, I asked Tony Jr. if I could go out with him to the parking lot and see it. He welcomed me to do so, and I was impressed with the perfection of the vehicle, which Tony Jr. had restored. I then returned to the apartment to continue my visit with Tony.

Tony Jr.'s car got Tony and I to talking about old cars, and I quickly discerned that this was a topic he loved. I asked Tony what kind of car he drives. It was pretty obvious he didn't still drive, but I phrased the question implying he still drives, to flatter him a bit.

"I have a Buick Riviera."

"Yeah? What year?"

"1991."

"Do you still drive?"

"No," Tony laughed.

Well, if he didn't drive anymore, maybe he would want to sell the car, and maybe at a bargain price.

"Are you going to sell the car?"

He didn't answer my question directly but instead invited me to take a look at it when I left and to tell me how much I thought it was worth. "It's a gray car and in perfect condition. It's parked along the side of the building right next to the street."

After I had been there for a little over an hour, I thanked Tony for allowing me to visit with him and asked if I could visit him again. He said that would be fine, but asked me to call first.

On the way out to my car, I marveled at what a nice man Tony is. Such a mellifluous voice! A marvelously friendly personality. This had to be the absolutely nicest man I had ever met. I remembered to walk past his car to take a look at it. It appeared to be, as Tony said, in mint condition. But I wasn't impressed. I already had a car. But maybe I would be interested in buying it if the price were right. How much was it worth? I had no idea. I wondered about his colon cancer, how bad it was.

Three Days Later

At 7:30 a.m. the phone rang. It was Tony. Why in the world was he calling me so early in the morning? After we exchanged pleasantries, he got right to the point.

"Did you look at my Buick Riviera?"

"Yeah, Tony, it's a very nice looking car. How much are you asking for it?" I began to fantasize that he would sell it to me for next to nothing.

"How much will you give me for it?"

He caught me totally off guard. How much would I give him for it? His question implied that I wanted the car very badly and was ready to make him an offer. Wait a minute. Tony had been a salesman all his life. This had to be a salesman's ploy: ask your prospective customer how much he would give you for his product. I felt myself starting to squirm. How was I going to get out of this? I was interested in his car only if he offered to sell it to me dirt cheap. But I had no idea of its worth on the open market.

"Tony, I tell you what. I can't make you an offer because I don't have a good feel for how much your car is worth. Let me do some research on what 1991 Buick Rivieras are selling for, and

I'll get back to you."

This satisfied him, and a few hours later I went to a nearby Buick dealer and talked to a salesman. Then I went to the village library and looked through several "red books" and "blue books" for prices of 1991 Buick Rivieras. My research showed that his car was worth from $3,000 to $7,000, depending on the condition. Assuming that Tony's car was in peak condition, it was worth near the higher price.

I called him back and told him about my research, that his car was worth $7,000 maximum, but that I wasn't prepared to offer him this much, since I already had two cars and just didn't want it badly enough. The most I would give him for it was the low end figure, $3,000. I expected him to hang up on me.

"Forget it. If that's all I can get for it, I'll give it to one of my daughters."

I felt terribly guilty for not buying his car, yet at the same time I felt good for researching it and for telling him the truth.

Two Days Later

I called Tony and asked if I could visit him on Wednesday, but he said no, that he was going to have company that day. At the time, Wednesday was the only day I could see him. Was he not wanting to see me because I wasn't buying his car?

A Week Later

I called Tony Jr. at his place of business to set up a visit with his dad, but he said to call his father directly. I then called his dad, and a woman, probably one of his daughters, answered, and after consulting Tony, told me he didn't want to talk right then. I told her I would call back tomorrow. Interesting. Did Tony not want to talk because he wasn't feeling well? Because of his car? Because of something I said or did on my first visit?

The Next Day

The hospice office called to inquire how I was doing with Tony. I said I had visited him once but had been rebuffed in two subsequent phone calls to try to arrange another visit. The office wasn't surprised, because Tony had become belligerent with his son and with two lady visitors. Tony, whom I thought was the nicest man I had ever met, get belligerent with anybody? I couldn't believe it. I said I would call him back and attempt another visit.

Minutes later I called Tony and asked if I could visit him again. He was very receptive, and we agreed that 11 a.m. Wednesday would be a good time.

The Next Day, Visit 2

At 10:55 a.m. I hiked up the flight of stairs and entered Tony's unlocked front door, calling out, "Hel-LOH-oooo."

"Come in," Tony sang out.

"It's Joe, the hospice volunteer," I yodeled. I entered Tony's bedroom and found him in bed resting comfortably. He appeared to be alone in his apartment. His son's bedroom door was closed.

I had told Tony on the phone that I was going to bring him some sunshine. I brought him a banana, a blooming cactus plant, and a handful of peppermint candies. He was very appreciative and had me give him one of the candies. He quickly removed the paper wrapper and put the candy in his mouth.

I complimented Tony on his salesmanship and the way he dealt with me about my possibly buying his car, coming out point blank and asking me how much I would give him for it. I told him he really had me squirming. He said he gave the car to his daughter Wilma. "But I told her she would have to give one-half of the car's value to her sister, Kay.

We talked about dogs. I told him I could have brought my daughter's new eight-week-old golden retriever to cheer him up. He said he likes dogs and owned one for many years.

I told Tony my two jokes about attorneys: (1) about heaven not having divorces, because there are no attorneys up there, and (2) about how to tell when an attorney is lying—when you see his lips move. He laughed heartily at both.

I wanted to ask Tony directly about his colon cancer but couldn't muster up the nerve. Instead, I asked him, jokingly, "How's your plumbing working, Tony?"

He laughed and said, "Fine." I let it go at that.

Tony told me he had had a heart attack about seven years ago and had bypass surgery and had a pacemaker/defibrillator installed. Just recently he had a doctor come in and deactivate the defibrillator. He no longer wanted to be revived if his heart should stop.

At 11:40 two ladies came into the apartment and into Tony's bedroom Tony introduced them to me: Shirley, a short, chubby lady of about 65 or so, began to sing, "Good morning to you, good morning to you, good morning dear Tony, good morning to you," to the melody of "Happy Birthday." The other lady introduced herself to me as Jane, Tony's sister-in-law.

The ladies' presence suddenly made me feel unwanted and unnecessary. I got up to leave and gracefully made my exit.

"I'll try to visit you, perhaps next Monday, Tony."

"Okay, Joe. Be sure and call first."

"Okay, Tony."

Walking to my car, I felt good. It was a great visit. We really communicated. I like Tony, and I was beginning to feel that he liked me. When I got home, I called the hospice office and left word on the tape recorder about my visit.

One Week Later, Visit 3

It was the day before Thanksgiving, and I called Tony at 10:40. He answered the phone, and

I told him I would like to visit him. He said he was tired. I said I just wanted to stop by for a moment and wish him a happy Thanksgiving. He said all right. I told him I would be there at about 11:15.

As soon as I got inside the front door at 11:05, I called out, "Hi, Tony, this is Joe, the hospice volunteer."

"Come on in, Joe," he replied in that rich, friendly voice.

I went into his bedroom, and he was lying on his back as usual. I thought he looked thinner than when I saw him last week. I reached down to shake his hand, and he had a firm grip. He told me to get a chair and to sit down. I went into the living room and brought back the little stuffed chair I had sat on last week. I again studied Tony's family picture, marveling at how handsome Tony and his son appeared and how beautiful his wife and two daughters looked.

I gave Tony a handful of hard peppermint candies and a big tangerine. He seemed pleased. He had me open one of the candies for him, and he put it in his mouth. I warned him that the tangerine had a lot of seeds. He asked to see it, and I handed it to him. He fondled it a bit and gave it back to me and I put it on his dresser. He said he loves tangerines and oranges.

We talked about Thanksgiving. Neither of us cares much for turkey. Tony said he likes chicken, pork, and roast beef; I said I like chicken a lot.

I asked if the two ladies who came last week were coming back today, and he said no, that his sister was coming this afternoon.

I told Tony about my accident in repairing my daughter's third-floor toilet. He laughed heartily. I had removed the toilet handle, turned and walked through the bathroom doorway to a nearby window to examine the handle closely. Still looking at the handle, I turned to return to the toilet and walked into the edge of the open bathroom door, bumping my forehead and cutting the back of my right hand twice on the handle latch. How I cut it twice, I still can't figure out. Then minutes later I stood up suddenly near the toilet and bumped my head on the slanted stucco ceiling. It was one of my worst days as a home handyman!

Tony said he had always been pretty good at fixing things around his house.

He said he had been a fisherman and hunter over the years, but recently gave his 20-guage shotgun to a grandson. I told him I had never owned a gun, because I was always fearful I might use it on somebody.

We discussed his being ill with colon cancer.

"This is a terrible way to have to die," he frowned.

I agreed with him with as much compassion as I could generate.

He said he wishes he could have died six years ago when he had his heart attack at age 78. We agreed that a heart attack would be a nice way to die. Go suddenly. I told him my father-in-law died of colon cancer when he was 70.

"How do you like using your portable potty (commode)?" I asked.

"Fine," he smiled.

"Would you like for me to empty it for you?"
The lid was down, and I wasn't sure if anything
was in it or not. I didn't smell anything.

"No, my son will do that."

"Do you still get up and go to the bathroom?"

"No. I use the commode."

"Are you in a lot of pain?"

"No."

"Are you taking morphine for pain?"

"No."

At 11:30 Tony's son came in the bedroom,
carrying a small bag of groceries. I noticed that
inside the bag were what I thought were
tangerines. He exchanged greetings with his dad
and with me, and then drifted off to the kitchen.

At 11:35 the front door opened and a feminine
voice said, "Hello."

"Who's that, Tony?" I asked.

"That's Robin. She's a nurse's aide. She's
come to give me a bath."

I stood up and greeted Robin, whom I had met
previously while visiting another hospice patient.

"Well, Tony, since you're going to get a bath, I
had better leave. Can I see you again next
Wednesday?"

"Sure, Joe. But call first."

I went into the kitchen and told Tony Jr. I
would drop in to visit his dad next week. He had
emptied his bag of groceries on the table, and I
saw the sack of tangerines.

"What a coincidence. I brought your dad a
tangerine," I laughed. "I warned him that it

contains a lot of seeds."

"I don't think the ones I bought have very many seeds," he said.

Heading out to my car, I thought about my bringing Tony a tangerine, and his son coming in from the store with a sack of tangerines. I wouldn't bring Tony anymore tangerines. But he likes the peppermint candy.

One Week Later, Visit 4

I called Tony at 10:25 and asked him if I could come over and visit him. With his consent, I arrived 20 minutes later. The temperature was in the low 40's, and it was a breezy, crisp morning with partly cloudy skies.

I went up the stairs and opened the door, calling out, "Tony, this is Joe."

"Come in, Joe."

I removed my jacket and placed it on the back of a sofa. Picking up a chair, I headed for Tony's room. I brought him some more peppermint candies in a small plastic bag, another tangerine (I changed my mind), and two Christmas tree angel ornaments. I set the candy and tangerine on his dresser and hung the angels, one around the head of a man in a little knickknack on a dresser on the right side of Tony's bed, and the other angel around one of two stags that Tony said he had bought in Toronto. He said they were made in Africa.

I showed Tony the Trappist monk brochure from Gethsemani, Kentucky, and told him how Dorothy (my wife) and I had visited there once. He had never heard of the Trappists. I told him how they make fudge, fruitcake, and cheese. "I'll send you some of their bourbon fudge." He said he wanted to pay me for it, but I told him, no, it was better to give than to receive. I asked him, that when the fudge comes, to at least taste it before giving it away. He promised he would.

He told me about his grandson Armand, who is 6 foot 4, and an airline pilot, and about his grandson Harry, who is 6 foot 6, who is learning how to be an airplane mechanic.

Tony reminded me that he originally had three sisters and four brothers, one of whom drowned at age 18. We talked again about my son being killed in a car wreck at age 16. I told him about my brother dying in a motorcycle accident at age 25, riding home from a Knights of Columbus meeting. I told him also about a member of my church choir dying from colon cancer at about age 40.

He told me he discovered he had colon cancer seven years ago after having a lower GI test. He declined surgery, which had been recommended, fearing that the surgery would spread the cancer to other parts of his body.

"The cancer still hasn't spread," Tony smiled.

I told Tony about my enlarged prostate and my surgery a year ago and how much the surgery had helped me.

A phone call from Tony's son interrupted our conversation. Tony said his son said to say hi to me.

Tony then had me leave the room, saying he wanted to get up and use his commode. I went out and closed the door and went into the living room and began studying the wall picture of Tony and his family taken years ago. The two daughters look so much like their mother, who is wearing earrings, has on a white dress and a fur coat. Tony Jr. has on a bow tie and a checkered top. Tony Sr. has on a bow tie and a double-breasted suit. I was struck how Tony was so handsome.

Pretty soon Tony called and said he was done, that I could come back in. When I opened his door, I expected to be greeted by a BM smell. I wasn't disappointed! It was pretty bad. But I remembered how bad my own smell was earlier this morning, and I endured Tony's without complaining.

"Does it smell in here?" Tony asked. He must have noticed the frown on my face.

"Yes, but it isn't that bad, Tony," I smiled. I offered to empty his commode for him, but he declined, saying there wasn't anything in it, that he had just passed gas.

Tony told me how when his 6-foot-6 grandson enters his room, he has to duck for the doorway. I stood up and compared my 5-foot-8 height to the doorway and estimated that, indeed, anyone 6 foot 6 really would have to duck.

"I think my mind is going," Tony said apologetically.

"No it isn't. Tony. You're still as sharp as a toothpick. You still look real healthy and appear to be only sixty-five."

"I've lost a lot of weight."

"How much do you weigh?"

"I don't know. I don't have a scale. But my skin is getting flabby."

Tony said he has a girlfriend, a widow. "It's the woman named Jane whom you met a few weeks ago when she came here. Her husband died of a heart attack when he was only forty-eight. She comes to see me once or twice a week."

Tony said he still has all his teeth, except for one. I was amazed.

"My dad died at age ninety with all his teeth."

"No he didn't!" I said. I couldn't believe it.

Tony told me he takes about five different kinds of medicines. He named two of them for me. Neither of us knew what they were for.

He told me he doesn't drink much beer, but that his favorite is a dark Irish beer. I laughingly told him how a Catholic nun friend, now in her 80's, still drinks a bottle or two of beer a day.

Robin, the nurse's aide, came at 11:45 to bathe Tony, and I prepared to make my departure.

"I've got Tony all ready for you, Robin," I joked.

I told Tony I would call him next week.

One Week Later, Visit 5

I called Tony at 10 o'clock, and he said I could come over right away for a visit. Before leaving home I prepared a small plastic bag of chocolates and mints and selected a tangerine for him. On the way I stopped at a liquor store with the intention of buying Tony some dark Irish beer, which he said was his favorite. Instead of Irish beer, I bought him a four-pack of Irish ale. My reasoning was: if Tony liked dark Irish beer, then he would like dark Irish ale even better. Tony couldn't remember the name of that dark Irish beer.

When I entered Tony's room, he was lying on his back holding his remote, watching what appeared to be a soap opera.

"Do you watch soap operas, Tony?"

"Sometimes."

"I watch very little TV, usually just news and sports," I told him.

Tony told me a joke: One day a rabbi went to this new barbershop to get a haircut, and the barber refused to take his money because he was a man of God. The next day a Protestant minister went to the same barber, who also refused his money because he, too, was a man of God. A day later a Catholic priest got a haircut and the same barber also refused his money because he too was a man of God. The next day six Catholic priests showed up at the barbershop to get a haircut.

Tony roared at his own joke. I laughed only slightly.

"The Catholic priests all wanted a free haircut. You get it?" He roared again. I couldn't help but laugh, not at the joke, but at the way Tony appreciated his own joke. I made a mental note to try and work up a better punch line.

I countered with my weather forecast joke. "Did you hear the terrible weather forecast?" I asked Tony.

"No," he looked at me with all seriousness.

"Chili today and hot tamale."

Tony laughed with gusto.

He had two boxes of chocolates on the dresser near his bed and invited me to help myself. I declined, saying it would make me fat.

"How much do you figure you weigh now, Tony?"

"Oh, I would guess maybe a hundred and fifty or a hundred and fifty-five. I used to weigh a hundred and seventy-five to a hundred and eighty in my prime."

"What did you have for breakfast?" I asked.

"Raisin toast, cereal, and coffee."

"Does your son fix your breakfast?"

"Yes. He usually fixes my lunch and brings it to me, too. My daughters or my girlfriend usually prepare my supper and bring it to me."

I couldn't help but think that Tony isn't anywhere near dying. He eats well, and he is mentally alert. He said he can make it out of bed okay to use his commode, but can't make it all the way to the bathroom.

"Is Robin, the nurse's aide, coming to bathe you today?"

"Yes. She's due here shortly. She comes on Monday, Wednesday, and Friday."

"Gee, maybe I should start coming on Thursday so my visit won't be interrupted by Robin."

"That would be all right."

"How do you like being on hospice, Tony?"

"It's all right." I was hoping for a more detailed reply, one that perhaps was full of deep feeling.

"What do you think about, knowing that you are on hospice with a relatively short time remaining to live."

"I don't mind that at all."

"Did you watch 'Tuesdays with Morrie' on TV?" I asked.

"No."

I explained that Morrie was a teacher dying of Lou Gehrig's disease.

"Our bishop died of Lou Gehrig's disease some years ago. His muscles gradually failed him, and the last to go were the muscles that controlled his eyelids. He communicated with his eyelids right up to the end."

"I saw Lou Gehrig and Babe Ruth play with the Yankees against the Sox at Sox Park. Babe Ruth was jealous of Gehrig. I saw Ruth hit some home runs," Tony boasted.

A knock on the front door and the door's opening and Robin's greeting of "Hello," announced her arrival to bathe Tony.

"You come on Monday, Wednesday, and Friday, don't you, Robin?"

"Yes."

"I think I'll start coming on Thursdays so you won't be interrupting my visit," I smiled. "It seems that I just get warmed up in getting Tony to talk when you come," I told her. When I left it was a little after 10:30.

One Week Later, Visit 6

I called Tony at about 10:30 and asked if I could come see him at about 2 o'clock. Tony said that would be fine and added that he remembered the name of the dark Irish beer, his favorite: Guiness. I told him I would bring him a bottle. He said to bring two: one for him and one for me.

I left my house at 1:30 and stopped at a liquor store and bought a six pack of Guiness dark Irish beer in bottles. Driving to Tony's, I debated with myself over how many bottles I would take to Tony. When I got there and parked, I decided to take only one bottle with me, for Tony, that if I drank a whole bottle, I might get too sleepy.

I entered Tony's apartment and was about to call out his name when a woman approached from his bedroom and looked at me questioningly.

"Yes?" she said.

I told her my name, and she said, "Oh, you're Joe. I've heard a lot about you from Tony. Come on in." She introduced herself as Kay, Tony's daughter. She said today is her birthday. I wanted to ask her age, but didn't have the courage.

Kay left Tony's room, and I entered. I detected a BM odor that on a scale of 1 to 10, I would categorize as about a 5.

Tony was lying in his usual position, on his back, with his head propped up on a couple of pillows. I greeted him and told him I had a bottle of Guiness beer for him. He asked me to have Kay open it and come back and at least taste it with him. I said okay and took the bottle to the kitchen, where Kay, after searching for about five minutes, found an opener and popped the cap. She gave me two small glasses, which I took into Tony's room along with the bottle of beer.

I poured some in a glass and gave it to him, and I poured some for myself in the other glass.

"To your health, Tony," I said, wondering if my words were appropriate. As I drank from my glass, I was amazed at the darkness of the beer. I tried to pour more beer into Tony's glass, but he declined and told me to drink the rest. I told him I had better not and took the unfinished bottle into the kitchen to Kay and suggested she put a small piece of plastic wrap over it and cap it with a rubber band. She tore off a piece of plastic and put it over the top and put the lid on over it and put it in the refrigerator. I congratulated her for her ingenuity.

I went back to Tony's room and sat down, and we enthused about how smooth and rich the beer tasted. He said the Irish drink a lot of the dark beer and then top it off with a good fight. I laughed and told him my wife's Irish father saw only three movies in his entire life: "The Quiet Man," "The Fighting 69th," and "Gone with the Wind."

Tony and I chatted for a bit, and he looked and acted very tired. The lights were off in his room, the blinds were drawn, and the TV was off. I told him I had better leave and let him sleep, and he agreed.

I went into the kitchen to chat with Kay about Tony. She was sitting at a table writing. I told her I didn't feel "useful" in visiting Tony the way I was doing, that I would like to start being "useful." She asked me what I meant by "useful."

"When I visit Tony, I just sit and talk with him. I don't do anything. If only I could do something for him during my visit. Or maybe if I could fill in for somebody, doing something for Tony."

"But you *are* being useful in doing just what you are doing," she said. "Just by visiting Tony, you *are* being useful."

So, just by my visits I was being useful to Tony? Hmmm, I hadn't looked at it that way. I guess, maybe, simply through my visits, I am being useful after all. Maybe she's right.

Kay said that in January her daughter is coming in from Europe and she wants to spend some time with her. I suggested maybe I could fill in for Kay somewhat with her dad while her daughter is here. She seemed to like this idea.

She said she comes in on most days at 1 o'clock and gives Tony lunch and stays with him until about 4 o'clock. I suggested I could come in at 1 o'clock next Wednesday and watch how she serves him lunch and maybe I could substitute for her sometime. She thought this was a good idea.

We chatted about another hospice volunteer, whose name is Wendy, who comes to see Tony on Mondays. Kay said shortly after I was assigned to begin visiting Tony, she had gone to see the hospice office and suggested perhaps it would be wise to have a woman volunteer visit Tony, that she thought Tony would be more receptive to a woman volunteer.

"I think Tony likes me. We seem to be getting along quite well," I assured her.

I told Kay about the "saga" of how I accidentally became a potential buyer for Tony's car, and how he had taught me a lesson in salesmanship by asking me how much I would offer him for the car, and how I was caught flabbergasted. I mentioned how I researched the value of the car on the open market and how I called Tony and explained I already had two cars and didn't much need a third, and I would have to offer him something near the low end of its worth (from $3,000 to $7,000), and that Tony then decided to give the car to his daughter, Wilma. I couldn't help but notice that Kay was very pretty.

Our conversation was interrupted by Tony calling her. I followed her into his room. He didn't seem to want much of anything but was just wondering what she was doing. I laughingly commented to Tony that Kay told me it was her birthday but that she wouldn't tell me how old she was. Tony immediately said, "Thirty-nine," and we all laughed.

I went up and shook Tony's hand warmly and told him I would see him next week.

On the way out to my car I thought about Tony's apparent overall health. He seemed to be very alert. I wondered about how his hand shook somewhat when he drank his beer. Kay had commented he had walked to the kitchen for lunch a few days ago, but it tired him out so much he later slept for four hours. Tony told me he has been having a pain in his left leg.

One Week Later, Visit 7

In preparing to visit Tony, I tied a Christmas ribbon around a bottle of Guiness Irish beer and put eight peppermint candies in a small plastic bag. I remembered to take along my hospice badge with my picture to show Kay I was a legitimate hospice volunteer.

I arrived at a few minutes before 1 o'clock expecting to meet Kay to help her fix lunch for Tony, but when I entered the unlocked door, I was met by Wilma, Kay's younger sister. She introduced herself and asked if I was Joe. She said she had given Kay the afternoon off and said Tony was asleep.

We went into the kitchen so I could help her fix Tony's lunch, but Tony called her, and I went with her to his room. Tony and I greeted each other, and Tony told Wilma he wanted to go to the bathroom. I left the room, and Tony actually got out of bed and walked to the bathroom by himself. I watched him walk from the bathroom to his room and was struck by how well he walked and by how skinny he looked.

When he got back in bed, Wilma combed his hair and had me sit in a chair on the right side of Tony's bed by his feet. Tony and I began to talk, and minutes later Wilma brought in his lunch: a sandwich on white bread with a peeled tangerine, which Wilma said was a clementine. I asked what was in the sandwich, and she said something that sounded like "brazoot." But when I got home, our daughter Jeanne told me he had probably said Prociuotto, a cheese she often buys at the supermarket. Tony wanted me to eat half of his sandwich, but I declined, and Wilma ate it. For Tony's beverage, Wilma gave him a small glass of dark wine.

Wilma sat down in a chair on the left side of Tony's bed by his feet, and the three of us began to chat. Wilma, her husband, their two sons, and their daughter live a few blocks from me. I told them I used to drop a girlfriend of one of our daughters off at a house on their street, and she said they were her neighbors, and she knew them well.

I told them about my Uncle Horace being divorced three times, but I screwed up the story. Rather than quote Horace as saying he had struck out the first time, struck out the second time, and then walked the third time, I said he had walked the first time, walked the second time, and struck out the third time. But they laughed heartily anyway.

Wilma said she remembers me from being in a singing group at out church. She said she and her husband used to go to the church regularly but stopped going after our pastor spoke of money one time too often.

I told Wilma I would return at 1 o'clock next Wednesday again if that would be okay, and she said it would be. I told her my plan to relieve Kay for a few days when her daughter comes in from Europe, and she said she would speak with Kay about this.

While I was there the phone rang and it was a friend of Wilma's, and Wilma was on the phone with her for half an hour or so. During that time I chatted with Tony about a wide range of topics, including the following:

- His being raised until he was nine in a little town in Oklahoma
- My traveling through Oklahoma City on a bus in the 1940's and how the bus station

had a rest room for Coloreds and one for whites. Tony remembered those days.

- The 1930's during the days of Prohibition, about Dillinger, Al Capone, Bugsy Siegel, and how "the lady in red" brought about the death of Dillinger. I told him how my wife's father had been a policeman during this time and had been written up in detective magazines of that era.

- Tony's health. He said he hardly has any pain at all. He said if he dared talk about the pain in his left leg, it would surely come about, and we laughed. He said he is having regular bowel movements and isn't discharging blood. I thought Tony's coloring was good, and he was always optimistic and upbeat.

Tony told me his father died at age 90, and when Tony went to the hospital to visit him, his dad was tossing pills in a wastebasket. Tony said he asked him what he was doing, and his quoted his father as saying, "These pills are bullshit."

Shortly after Wilma finished her phone call with her girlfriend, her brother, Tony Jr., called, and their conversation lasted about five minutes. Then someone else called, and that conversation lasted another five minutes.

They gave me a small wrapped Christmas package, which I opened before I left. It was a Santa Claus tree ornament.

Tony appeared to be falling asleep, so I shook his hand, and Wilma walked me to the door, and I shook her hand. She said she teaches art and has hobbies of jewelry-making and ceramics. On the way out I spoke highly of the beautiful family portrait. I left at 2:40, and had been there for an hour and 40 minutes. It was a great visit.

When I got home I gave the Christmas ornament to Dorothy to hang on our tree.

One Week Later, Visit 8

When I arrived at 12:55, Wilma was in her father's bedroom checking on him as he was finishing his lunch. She had gone out to lunch with her husband and had brought Tony some of their lunch. The dishes on Tony's tray were empty, and Wilma was removing them.

I placed my jacket on the sofa in the living room and went into the bedroom. Seeing the chair near the other side of the foot of the bed, I went over to it and sat down. I thought Tony once again looked good, but his hair seemed a bit unruly. After Wilma got his dishes taken into the kitchen, she sat down on the chair by the other side of the foot of the bed.

Minutes later Tony asked her if she would give him a haircut. She agreed, and launched into the somewhat intricate task of having Tony get out of bed and sit on a chair. Tony apparently had his pajama bottoms off, and Wilma held up a blanket so Tony could swing his feet off the bed and sit up and put his pajama bottoms on. Then Tony said, "Okay, I'm decent. You can put the blanket down now."

Wilma helped her father onto the chair, which she had moved close to the bed. I remained where I was. Wilma proceeded with the haircut using a razor blade shaver to shave his neck, and scissors and comb, which she handled deftly. I complimented her on the nice job she was doing, which she really was. When she was done, Tony's haircut looked quite professional. I kidded Tony that she was giving him a crew cut.

I took out a copy of a newsletter from a priest friend and read them the part where he said his church "sleeps" 300. They laughed. Wilma knew the priest, too, and we talked of his frequent travels. She asked where the priest had been traveling to, and I told her his letter said he had been given a ticket to London, and went to London and then flew to Ireland to visit with relatives and friends. We talked about how the priest used to go on a couple of cruises a year as ship's chaplain and come back tanned and say, "Well, somebody has to do it."

I told them I was going to bring along my grandchildren's "Knock, Knock" book, but I thought I had better not, lest Tony might throw me out. They laughed.

We talked about the price of haircuts back in the old days. Tony and I both could remember when they cost 25 cents. Wilma said when she first started taking her sons to the barbershop they cost $2.

I kidded Tony, complimenting him that he was going to make it to the next millennium. We chatted about the millennium, as to whether it begins January 1, 2000, or January 1, 2001.

After Wilma finished giving Tony his haircut, she asked him to take off his top so she could take it outside and shake it to remove the hair. I complimented Tony on his physique, and he said he used to have a nice build when he was young.

When Tony got back in bed after his haircut, he moaned and groaned something awful. I told him I could feel his pain. I asked him where it hurt, and he said, "All over."

I asked Tony if we dared talk about the pain in his left leg lest the pain start to return, and he smiled and said, "Let's don't talk about it."

I reminded Wilma I could stay a while in the afternoon with Tony when Kay's daughter comes in from Europe. She said she would tell Kay.

Wilma opened the window a little bit in Tony's room, after first asking her dad if she could do so. The room cooled off nicely. The room always seemed so hot. Suddenly a bad smell was wafting my way, and I was wishing I could get up and move. But I stayed where I was, and the smell went away. After Tony complained of feeling cold, Wilma shut the window, but not quite all the way, so just a tiny bit of air could still come in.

The weather outside was nice: sunny, in the 40's, but breezy.

I didn't take Tony any gifts today. I noticed he still had his two little sacks of peppermints I had brought during other visits.

We talked about restaurants, and Wilma said there's a real nice Italian restaurant at Broad Street and Charleston.

Wilma scratched Tony's back after he asked her to.

We had a nice visit, and before I knew it, it was 2:20, when Tony said he was getting sleepy. So I said good-bye, and shook his hand and left.

One Week Later, Visit 9

At a few minutes before 1 o'clock, I chortled, "Hello!" I didn't hear a reply and sang out another announcement of my presence.

Then I heard Tony respond faintly, "Joe?"

I went into his bedroom, and he was in bed as usual. Neither Kay nor Wilma was there. I asked him who gave him lunch, and he said Robin (the nurse's aide) did. "You could have given me a call, and I would have been happy to fix your lunch, Tony," I told him. Tony said to bring in a chair and sit down and visit with him.

"Well, Tony, we made it into the new millennium, didn't we?"

We laughed.

"Say, I brought along a senior citizens' paper that has some classified ads for both men and women looking for companionship. You and I ought to place an add in there, Tony," I laughed.

I read him four or five of the entries from women, and then a couple of the entries from men. He began to get into the spirit of the thing and seemed to get a kick out of it.

"My wife, Dorothy, prepared an ad for me," I said. "Here it is: 'White Catholic, 70, bald, short, homely, hates movies, dislikes eating out, controlling, seeks widow with similar tastes, must be rich, beautiful, and sexy.'"

I thought Tony would die laughing.

We chatted about odds and ends. He spoke about his girlfriend, Jane, who he said is 82, and is his sister-in-law.

At 1:45 the phone rang, and Tony started to chat with someone who sounded like an old friend. I stepped out of his bedroom and sat in the living room until he was done, about 10 minutes later. I returned to his bedroom, and we chatted for about 10 minutes when he said he felt like napping.

I left at 2:05. He said 1 p.m. Wednesday is a good time to visit him. I told him I'd see him next week.

One Week Later, Visit 10

The weather was partly cloudy, the temperature was 36, and a light breeze was from the northeast. Planes were landing into the wind toward the airport. At a few minutes before 1 o'clock, I walked right in, calling out, "Hello!"

"Joe?"

"Yeah, this is Joe."

I went in and put my sack of goodies on Tony's dresser.

"What do you have?" he asked.

"It's a secret," I said.

I turned and went into the living room to remove my coat and put it on the sofa and returned with a chair to Tony's bedroom.

Tony asked me to fill his plastic drinking container, telling me to go into the kitchen and let the water run until it was cold. He said Robin had filled it for him but didn't let the water run long enough, that the water was warm.

I went into the kitchen with the container and

118

was amazed at how warm the water was out of the tap. I let it run for about five minutes until it was cold. The kitchen faucet had one of those water purifier units on it. I wondered if it did any good. I filled his container and took it in to Tony and sat down.

I showed him what I had in the bag: a book on the origins of words and phrases, a book with 1,000 knock-knock jokes, and an issue of *Guideposts*. I asked Tony if I could read him some stuff, and I read him a few short things from *Guideposts*, a few items from the origin of words and phrases, and three knock-knock jokes. Neither of us could stand any more knock-knock jokes, so I stopped.

He received a phone call, and it was Elmer, calling from an apartment on the ground floor across the atrium. He had called to tell Tony he wanted to give him some homemade oxtail soup. Tony sent me over to get it.

Elmer was practically bald, wore gold-rimmed glasses, and was several inches shorter than I. He had a birdcage with two birds in it. I asked him how old he was, and he said 83, "a year younger than Tony." I told him I was the kid on the block. He said, "That's right. That's why we're sitting down and you're doing the running." I laughed.

I went into his kitchen and watched him spoon out some soup into a little plastic dish and press a lid on it. I told him not to put it in a sack, that I could carry it hot. And the container was hot! I could barely hold it. I kept switching it from hand to hand as I hurried back to Tony's apartment, wishing I would have let him put it in a sack.

Tony had me put the soup in his refrigerator. I wrote my name and phone number down for Tony, and he put it in his night stand drawer. I told him to tell Kay to call me if I could be of any help while her daughter is here from Europe.

Tony said he was getting tired and about to fall asleep. So I left. It was 1:50.

One Week Later, Visit 11

The hospice office called on Monday and left word I should give Tony his lunch today. I called Tony at 10 o'clock and told him what she said. "My lunch has already been set out for me: a sandwich and a beverage," he told me.

I acted surprised and suggested I come over at noon and have lunch with him. I wondered who got their signals mixed up concerning preparing Tony's lunch.

"That would be fine, Joe. I think Robin (the nurse's aide) will be done with me by then."

At a few minutes before noon, Robin had just finished giving Tony his bath. Tony was in the bathroom with the door closed. I chatted briefly with Robin, and she said Tony was her seventh patient of the day, that she was now done and was heading home to do her housecleaning and take care of her daughter.

As Robin was busy cleaning up, Tony called from the bathroom asking for her to come in and assist him. She went in, and I went into the kitchen and killed a few minutes and came out. Robin was then in the bedroom with Tony.

"Has Tony been behaving himself?" I asked Robin.

"Tony always behaves himself," she laughed.

A few minutes later Robin left, and I asked, "Are you ready for your lunch, Tony?"

"Yes."

I brought in a chair and sat down and we started to eat our lunch. Tony had a ham and cheese sandwich, a small glass of red wine, and an orange. He ate from a portable tray as he sat up in bed. I had a cup of hot tea from my Thermos, a peanut butter-jelly sandwich, some lettuce and slices of tomato, and a tangerine.

"Who fixed lunch for you, Tony?"

"My son fixed it for me before he left for work." Apparently one of Tony's daughters had called the hospice office thinking that no one was going to fix Tony's lunch.

We had a spirited conversation while we ate.

"I haven't moved my bowels for three days."

"You haven't? Do you have any suppositories? They ought to bring on a BM."

He said he had some, and I suggested he give himself one, that maybe it would help him move his bowels.

Tony said his granddaughter from Europe and her son stopped by twice to visit with him.

Soon Tony seemed to be getting sleepy, and I excused myself and left. It was 1 o'clock. I had been there for slightly more than an hour.

Two Days Later, Visit 12

The hospice office called to talk to me about Tony, saying that Tony had hurt Kay's feelings, that Kay refuses to sit with him anymore. I was asked to sit with Tony two days a week instead of one. I said I would give it a try. Of course, Wendy, another hospice volunteer, was visiting Tony on Mondays. That would make three hospice volunteer visits a week.

Five Days Later, Visit 13

I phoned Tony at 10 o'clock and asked him if I could come over at noon and eat lunch with him. Sure, he told me.

At a few minutes before 12, Tony greeted me as usual and told me a nurse's aide was coming at 12. So we held off eating lunch, and at 12:10 Sonja, a nurse's aide, arrived. I went into the kitchen so she could begin giving Tony his bath.

I wasn't a happy camper as I sat at the kitchen table. Hadn't I called Tony to see if I could come over at noon and have lunch with him? And hadn't Tony said yes, without mentioning that a nurse's aide was coming at noon to give him a bath? So, here I was, sitting in his kitchen waiting for him to have his bath! Oh, brother! Beginning to get hungry, I ate my lunch: a peanut butter-jelly sandwich, a pear, and a cup of hot tea from my Thermos. I hadn't brought anything to read, and began to read anything I could get my hands on: the label on Tony's wine bottle, the label on a nearby box of cereal, and other food labels. I began to saunter about the kitchen, examining various objects and pictures on the wall. I looked out the kitchen window across the street at the funeral home and its parking lot, wondering if that was where Tony would be taken when he died.

Finally at 12:45 Sonja left. She had been here for a little more than half an hour, but it had seemed like an eternity. I went back into Tony's room and explained to him I just got too hungry and ate my lunch without him. I chatted with him while he ate the ham and cheese sandwich and drank the small glass of red wine his son had left for him.

"How are those bowels doing, Tony? I remember you had told me they hadn't been moving like they were supposed to."

"Too much," he laughed. "I was up all night. They gave me a laxative or something to make them move. And boy, did they move!"

I had told the hospice office that Tony had said his bowels hadn't moved for three days. The office said if a blockage occurred, the patient would get nauseous, that nothing would go down. Tony couldn't have had a blockage: he wasn't nauseous, and his sandwich and wine went down just fine.

I left when Tony said he was getting sleepy. It was about 1:30.

Three Days Later, Visit 14

At 11:55, bringing my lunch: cheese, tomato, and onion sandwich, three kiwis that I had peeled and cut up, and a cup of hot tea from my Thermos, I found Tony practically asleep, responding feebly when I called him from the front door. I hadn't phoned first, wanting to take a chance and just see what would happen. I took off my jacket, hat, and gloves and went into his bedroom. He was lying on his back and looked very sleepy.

"Did I wake you up, Tony?"

"Yes, but that's all right."

"I brought some food so I could have lunch with you."

"Oh, I'm sorry, Joe. I just finished my lunch. Robin was here and fixed it for me. But go ahead and sit down and eat your lunch and we can talk." I brought in a chair and proceeded to eat. We chatted about a lot of things, including the following:

- His granddaughter and her son went back to Europe.
- We decided that the little Cuban boy who was so prominent in the news would be better off staying with relatives in the United States.
- I told him about the Korean War, how the battlefield had seesawed back and forth.

He told me a joke about an Irishman who had a bottle of whiskey and used to take a sip from it every day. One day he looked at the amount of whiskey remaining in the bottle and thought that someone had snitched a drink. Each day he began marking the bottle at the whiskey level. Finally he decided to get even with the thief. He urinated in the bottle and again marked the level. The next day he looked at the mark. Sure enough. Someone had drunk from the bottle, but whoever it was had attached a note that read: "I don't know what you did to this whiskey, but it sure tastes good. Can I have the recipe?"

I snickered a bit at the joke. It was dumb, but

it was also funny.

"I told it to Wendy on Monday, and she laughed real hard," Tony said.

Tony said his father and his father's brother had settled in Illinois, but went to work in a coal mine in Oklahoma, where Tony was born.

At a few minutes after 1 o'clock I said good-bye to Tony, telling him I would see him Friday.

Four Days Later, Visit 15

I had called first to alert Tony I was coming, after having asked the hospice office if I should continue visiting Tony twice a week. I was told, yes. At 11:55, bringing my lunch: peanut butter and jam with a sliced onion, three kiwis that I had peeled and cut up, some crisp green lettuce, and a cup of hot tea in my Thermos, I walked in and announced myself, and Tony invited me in. I brought a chair into his bedroom, along with my lunch, and greeted him and sat down. He had me help him get started with his lunch. His son had left him a dish of tuna from a can and what appeared to be a piece of bread or a biscuit in a little plastic sack. Tony had me go into the kitchen and get him a glass of wine. I came back with the wine in a rather large glass, and Tony said it was too much. I went back and returned with the wine in a smaller glass, and Tony approved.

We started eating our lunches and conversing. I brought along a joke book and told Tony a joke or two that I had just read from the book. I read him a couple of jokes, which he liked.

Tony told me that when he was a boy, probably about six or seven, he was struck in his right eye with an arrow that a neighborhood boy had shot, which blinded the eye. Ever since, Tony has had vision only in his left eye. He said the loss of an eye never bothered him.

Sometimes I will attempt to do things with one hand covering one of my eyes just to try to comprehend how people with one-eye vision do it. It amazed me that Tony said having vision in only one eye never bothered him.

Right after we finished lunch, Robin (nurse's aide) arrived to give Tony his bath. So I made my departure.

Two Days Later, Visit 16

I called Tony at 9:45 to remind him I would be coming over at 12 o'clock to have lunch with him. He seemed glad for my phone call and that I was coming.

I arrived at 11:45, thinking it wouldn't hurt to get there a bit early. I was greeted by Tony's son. He told me some melted snow on the roof had leaked through the concrete ceiling into their second-floor apartment. I looked up and could see water stains along one of the concrete support beams.

"The worst part of it is that the water came down on my clothes," he said.

"When did it happen?" I asked.

"Two days ago."

"That's funny," I said, "as I was walking from my car just now, I looked up at the tops of these

126

apartment buildings and noticed that they all had a flat roof and that there were no icicles hanging down. Flat roofs are prone to leaking."

"I guess the freezing and thawing and that recent heavy snow backed water up from the rain gutter. I called the apartment owner and he sent someone up there to check it out."

"Gee, that's too bad the water leaked onto your clothes," I said, trying to sound compassionate.

"Our apartment is starting to smell real musty with all that water. And my poor clothes!"

"Is Robin here?" I asked.

"Yeah. She's almost done."

"How's your dad doing?"

"Well, he said he's not too interested in eating his lunch, because his bowels haven't been moving."

With that, Tony Jr. went into the bedroom to say good-bye to his dad and to Robin. I could see Robin scurrying about. I decided to remain in the living room until she left. Tony Jr. left and Robin came through the living room saying I could go into the bedroom now, that she was done.

I took my lunch into the bedroom, greeted Tony, and sat down. He was just starting his lunch. His plate appeared to have a full-course meal on it: a meat dish, corn, and green beans. His usual small glass of wine was on his tray.

As Tony proceeded to eat, I remembered his son had told me Tony probably wouldn't eat much lunch, but he seemed very interested and ate it all. I asked him if his bowels were blocked again, and he muttered that yes, they were. I said he probably should get back onto that medicine that opened up his bowels the last time, and he agreed.

I had brought my joke book with me but told Tony I would hold off reading him some more jokes until I finished my lunch. I had brought another peanut butter-jelly sandwich, some lettuce, a tomato, and my Thermos of hot tea. When I finished eating, I read him about a dozen jokes, and he seemed to appreciate each one. His typical response was a brief laugh and the comment, "That's cute."

We started talking about chop suey, and Tony said it means "leftovers" in Chinese.

Finally his eyelids began to droop and he told me he was feeling drowsy. He apologized, saying he couldn't help it, but his brain just shut down. I gave him my farewell greetings and left. I told him I would see him Friday, if that was okay with him.

On my way to my car, I thought Tony looked good. He was alert and in good spirits.

Five Days Later, Visit 17

I called at 9:30 and asked Tony if he would like me to have lunch with him. Yes, he said. I arrived at 11:50. The weather was about 25 degrees, breezy, and sunny. Planes were approaching the airport from the southwest, with their flight path just to the west of his apartment.

I picked up a chair and brought it into Tony's room. We were all set for lunch, except for Tony's wine. I went to the kitchen and poured him a small glass of his Livingstone burgundy. Tony's son had left him a ham sandwich and an orange. I had brought a three-decker peanut butter/jelly sandwich, some kale, and a cup of hot tea in my Thermos.

The minute I sat down I told Tony I could tell that Robin (nurse's aide) hadn't been there yet because the blanket was hanging way down on his left side. After Robin leaves, the blanket is always straight. Also, Tony's room had a bad odor, probably from a dirty diaper. After Robin leaves, his room always smells good. I didn't want to mention anything about the smell.

It seems we had barely started eating when Robin came in the front door and announced herself. I moved my lunch into the kitchen, leaving Robin to commence with Tony's bath.

In the kitchen, I finished my lunch and catnapped. I went to the window and looked out at the parking lot of the funeral home across the street. I made a mental note to ask Tony if this was the funeral home of his choice. I watched a few planes heading toward the airport. I studied a wall picture of Tony Jr. taken when he was in the military.

After a while Robin came into the kitchen to refill Tony's drinking glass, letting the water run for a long time to get it cool. She said she was done, that I could go back to his room. After Robin left, Tony and I started talking again. He finished his ham sandwich, and I offered to peel his orange for him, but he declined and peeled it himself.

I read him a dozen or so jokes from my joke book, and he laughed pretty hard at each. I told him I didn't want to tell him any dirty jokes, and he agreed he didn't want to hear any. I told him that when I went to a book store to select a joke book to read to him, that the first one I looked at seemed to have all dirty jokes.

I asked Tony the name of the funeral home across the street from his apartment, and he said he didn't know.

"After you die, will you be taken there?" I asked with some trepidation.

"I don't know," he shrugged, as if the question were unimportant.

"You want them to surprise you, huh?" I laughed.

"Yeah," Tony joined my laughter.

"What do you think awaits a person when he dies?" Tony asked, with all seriousness.

His question caught me by surprise. "I've read a lot about what happens, but I just don't know, I guess," I muttered. I was tempted to give him the standard Catholic interpretation as I remembered it from my catechism classes, but decided not to.

"You know, Joe," Tony said, "I've got my doubts about all this heaven and hell stuff. I think when you die, it's all over."

I didn't feel it appropriate to dispute Tony on this. After all, I wasn't his chaplain.

"I think you told me during one of my visits that you will be buried next to your wife, didn't you?"

"Yes."

"Do you have any preference for either a conventional burial or a cremation?" I asked.

"No."

"Let them surprise you, huh?"

We laughed, and then I asked Tony to guess how much it cost me to have my muffler/tailpipe replaced.

"Oh, I'd guess maybe $250."

"Would you believe, $600?"

Tony shook his head in disbelief.

We continued chatting until Tony started getting drowsy. I left at 1:40.

One Week Later, Visit 18

I called Tony at 9:45 to remind him I was coming over to have lunch with him, that is, if he wanted me to. He said to come on over. I told him I would see him at about noon.

It was about 45 degrees, sunny, with no wind, and melting snow at 11:55 when I called out to Tony as I entered his apartment.

"Hi, Joe," he responded. He sounded in good spirits.

I went into his bedroom, carrying with one hand my plastic bag bearing my lunch and two books, and with the other hand, the chair from Tony's living room. Tony said Robin hadn't arrived yet. I already discerned that: from the disheveled blanket on his bed and from the slightly bad odor in the room. We both figured we should start our lunch, and if Robin came to start his bath, I would go into the kitchen and wait for her to finish.

Tony told me that Wendy, the other hospice volunteer who sees him on Mondays, was very upset.

"She told me she was having a fireplace installed by three workmen, and after they left the other day, she noticed some of her jewelry missing. I told her not to be upset about this, that she has to get over it."

"I still haven't met Wendy," I told Tony. "I attend most of the hospice volunteer meetings, and I've yet to see her there."

Tony's lunch consisted of a dish of tuna, a biscuit, tangerine, and his usual small glass of burgundy wine. I was eating my peanut butter-strawberry jam-chopped onion sandwich, lettuce, and drinking a cup of hot tea from my Thermos. We made pleasant small talk as we ate.

When we finished eating, I read him about a dozen jokes from my joke book. Before I left home, I read a number of them, marking about eight I thought were funny. After I read those to him, which he enjoyed, I read him about half a dozen more. Then I switched to reading items from the other book I brought, dealing with trivia items. He didn't seem to enjoy these, so I went back to the joke book.

Tony interrupted me to tell me a joke he said he had heard recently. As soon as he started to tell it, I recognized it as one I had read to him the week before. But I didn't say anything and laughed when he finished. It was the one about the Pope going for a boat ride with a friend. Out on the lake the Pope's hat blows off into the water, and the Pope gets out of the boat and walks across the water, retrieves his hat, and gets back into the boat. "Gee, I didn't know you couldn't swim," the other fellow says.

While Tony was eating, he had me do a few small tasks for him: get him a paper towel three times, get him a toothpick, carry his dishes into the kitchen, refill his water bottle with cool water from the kitchen, making sure to let the water run a while until it was cool.

I asked Tony if he was having any pain, and he said no, but he was having difficulty keeping awake. I offered to take him for a walk, as I had offered before, in all seriousness, but he declined.

Pretty soon Tony's eyelids began to droop, so I decided to leave. "Say, Tony," I said getting up to leave, "where did you say you kept your jewelry?" We both laughed and said our good-byes.

Walking to my car, I passed Robin heading for Tony's apartment.

"Hi, Robin."

"Hi, Joe. I'm running late today," she confessed. I was thankful. I had had a real nice uninterrupted visit with Tony.

One Week Later, Visit 19

I called Tony at 10 o'clock to remind him I was coming for lunch. When I arrived at 11:50, the sky was clear, the temperature 30 degrees, and a slight breeze was from the northeast, so planes were landing from the southwest toward the airport.

Tony was alone, and I walked into his bedroom carrying my sack bearing my lunch, Thermos, joke book, and some reading material just in case I had to wait in the kitchen while Robin bathed him.

Tony's blanket was hanging down at an angle.

"You know how I can tell Robin hasn't been here yet?" I said.

"How?"

"When your blanket is nice and straight, that tells me Robin was just here. Since the corner of your blanket is hanging down, that tells me Robin hasn't arrived yet."

"She just left," Tony laughed.

"She just left? No kidding! Jeez, there goes my theory!" We both laughed. "Here, let me straighten that blanket out for you." I went around to the other side of his bed and evened out the blue quilt.

"What were you doing to mess up your blanket like that, Tony?" Tony joined me in laughing.

We exchanged pleasantries, and I sat down and poured myself a cup of my hot tea and started to eat my three-decker peanut butter-strawberry jam sandwich. Tony had already eaten his lunch, even though I had reminded him on the phone two hours earlier I was coming. I took his empty dish and empty wine glass into the kitchen. He said the dish had contained spaghetti. The bit that remained looked appetizing.

I told Tony a few simple jokes while I ate. Midway through my lunch his son came in bearing a few bags of groceries. He spoke to his father, and I thought his son sounded a bit snappish. His father asked Tony Jr. to "call Peggy (hospice nurse) and tell her my laxative medication needs adjusting, that it's a bit too powerful and keeps me up most of the time going to the bathroom." His son said he would call her. Minutes later his son came back into the bedroom and said good-bye and left.

I finished my lunch and read Tony about a dozen jokes I had read and marked as funny before I left home. He enjoyed most of them. Then he started getting drowsy, and I prepared to leave.

"Do you want me to come for lunch Friday?" I asked him.

"Yes, that would be nice," he said.

"Is Robin coming Friday?"

"No, she has off for a few days."

I asked Tony if I could take him for a walk, and he said no. I asked him if he is getting up and going to the bathroom, and he said he is using the commode near his bed.

Two Days Later

I called Tony at about 10 o'clock to remind him I was coming over to have lunch with him. He apologized and said his sister and girlfriend were coming over, that I shouldn't come.

Five Days Later, Visit 20

I tried calling Tony four or five times between 10 and 10:45, and each time he did not answer the phone. I could not leave a message, as he did not have an answering recorder. Considerably worried, I called the hospice headquarters. The people I knew there were not in, so I left a message on a tape recording, asking if something had happened to Tony.

I then called Tony's son and told him his father wasn't answering the phone, and he became quite concerned and said he would go over there right away. He called me back about 15 minutes later and said everything was okay, that he had forgot to leave the phone by his father's bed. He let me talk to his dad, and I told Tony I would be coming over at noon.

At 11:50, I went into his bedroom, carrying the chair and my sack containing my Thermos of hot tea, a tomato, and my peanut butter/strawberry jam/chopped-onion sandwich. A slight odor, as though Tony's diaper needed changing, told me Robin had not arrived yet.

Just as I sat down, Tony asked me to go into the kitchen and fix him some lunch. At first he asked for soup, then changed his mind, asking for a Thomas bun and locks and cream cheese. I found the cream cheese and the bun, and brought those in and told Tony I couldn't find the locks. I went back into the refrigerator and found a container of smoked salmon and brought that to Tony. He said those weren't locks, but they would be okay. Tony disappointedly said the bun was cold. Just as he was about to put cream cheese on it, Robin entered the front door. Tony had me take everything back into the kitchen, and he said I should go into the kitchen and eat my lunch.

I went into the kitchen and toasted his bun and spread cream cheese on it and put a slice of smoked salmon on each half and left it on a plate on the kitchen table. I sat down and ate my sandwich and drank my cup of hot tea from my Thermos. As I ate, I read over some more jokes that I could read to Tony.

Just as Robin was finishing with Tony, his son walked in. He said he came home to have lunch because he had to interview a woman who was going to sit with his father this weekend when he wouldn't be home. Tony Jr. looked at what I had fixed his father and said his dad would rather have the locks. He opened the refrigerator and got out a package of locks, which he explained was almost like raw salmon that had been partially smoked. He spread some more cream cheese on the bun, saying his dad liked a lot of cream cheese. Then he took out a slice and put it on a bun and put a lid on it. It looked and smelled delicious. Hey, Tony has good taste!

Tony Jr. put the chunks of smoked salmon back in the plastic bag with what had remained of the package I had opened. He sat down at the table, and I asked him if he eats the almonds that were in a package on the table. "Yes, because they're rich in vitamins."

Robin came into the kitchen saying she was done with Tony. I took the plate bearing the bun, cream cheese, and locks into Tony and returned to the kitchen, and Tony Jr. poured a small glass of wine for his dad. It wasn't the dark burgundy, but was a light wine. I asked Tony what it was, but he said he didn't know.

When Robin left, I gave Tony his lunch, which he thoroughly enjoyed. I told him about the scandal at an area Catholic church involving the pastor. Tony said he had already heard about it from his daughter Wilma.

137

"I think all Catholic priests are queers," Tony confided. His statement caught me by surprise, and I couldn't help but laugh, although I knew that on the face of it, his statement was incorrect. Not "all" priests fit that category, only "some."

After I read Tony a half dozen or so jokes, his son sat down on the living room sofa and turned on the TV, watching whatever, waiting for the lady to show up who was going to interview to sit with his father over the weekend. Then I heard a female voice talking to Tony Jr., and his father and I concluded it must be the lady who was going to sit with him.

I told Tony I was all done reading him jokes and said good-bye. I had to go into the kitchen to get my sweater, which I had draped over a kitchen chair, the one on which Tony Jr. was sitting.

"Excuse me, Tony, but I have to get my sweater," I said, noticing that a lady was sitting opposite him at the table.

She said, "Hi, Joe," and I didn't recognize her.

"How did you know my name?" I asked her. "Do I know you?"

"Yes. I'm Kay, Tony's daughter."

I was embarrassed. I hadn't recognized her.

Then we made small talk about the pastor and about her daughter coming in from Europe to visit. I told her I was disappointed when she didn't call me to help out while her daughter was here.

Just as I was heading for the door to leave, a lady walked in and identified herself as Gertrude, the woman who was coming to interview to sit with Tony over the weekend. I glanced at my watch as I headed for my car. It was 1:10.

Two Days Later, Visit 21

I called Tony at 10:30 to remind him I would be over at noon to have lunch with him. He told me his family had left an artichoke for his lunch. An artichoke? Wow! I wondered what the occasion was.

At 11:50, I went into his room; the tray was over his bed, and a dish containing the remnants of an artichoke was on the tray.

"Hey, Tony, you ate without me."

"Robin was here and she warmed it up for me," he apologized.

"I can always tell when Robin has been here, because your bed cover is straight," I laughed.

I cleared up Tony's dirty dishes and sat down and ate my peanut butter/strawberry jam/chopped-onion sandwich and drank the hot tea from my Thermos. I was disappointed that Tony had already eaten his artichoke. I was going to kid him about it.

One of the things we chatted about was the afterlife.

"I'm not sure if there is a God or not, or a heaven or a hell," he confided. "When I die, if there's a God and a heaven, I think I'll get to heaven, because I've always tried to do what is right." I believed him and momentarily pictured myself as the Supreme Being welcoming Tony into heaven.

I read Tony a couple dozen jokes from my joke book. As I was getting ready to leave, Tony said Gertrude was coming at 8 o'clock tonight to stay with him over the weekend while his son was in Wisconsin.

"Hey, Tony," I whispered, "I glanced at Gertrude as I was leaving Wednesday, and she wasn't bad looking! You better behave yourself this weekend!"

"Why should I?" he smiled. We roared with laughter.

Two Weeks Later, Visit 22

I called Tony at 9:45 to tell him I was coming at noon to have lunch with him. At 11:50, our lunch was interrupted by Robin's arrival to bathe him. After waiting in the kitchen, I returned to Tony's room and read him a couple dozen jokes. I told him I would return on Friday to have lunch with him.

Two Days Later, Visit 23

I decided not to call Tony ahead of time as I usually do, to sort of test his memory. I had told him Wednesday I would be returning today to have lunch with him. At 11:50, Tony expressed surprise at my visit. He had forgot I was coming and told me two lady friends were due at noon to have lunch with him. He totally flunked my memory test!

I proceeded to read him a few jokes, waiting for them to arrive. I got about half way into a joke when Robin came to bathe him. Since Tony said two lady friends were coming to have lunch with him, I decided to leave.

Lesson learned: be sure to call Tony before leaving home and remind him I am coming.

Five Days Later, Visit 24

At exactly noon, Robin, the nurse's aide, was bathing Tony. From the living room I called out, "Hello."

"Hello, Joe," Tony replied.

"I'm almost done," Robin said.

"I'll go sit in the kitchen until you finish, Robin."

I sat down at the kitchen table and started reading my joke book, which I had brought to read to Tony. Robin finished with Tony at 12:25, and I went into his bedroom and sat down and we began eating our lunch. Tony had a sandwich and small glass of wine that had been left for him by his son. I had brought along some leftovers: grilled cheese sandwich, hot dog, and some hot tea.

We made some warm and friendly conversation as we ate. He was alert and ate all of his sandwich and drank all of his wine.

"Hey, Tony. You're going to be eighty-five tomorrow, aren't you?"

"Yes," he smiled.

"Tell me, what is the secret of your longevity."

"Just staying alive," he laughed.

"Is your family going to give you a party?"

"I don't know."

Getting off the subject, I asked him if he had been walking to the bathroom or using the commode near his bed. "I walk to the bathroom only when someone is around to help me. Otherwise, I use the commode."

I began reading jokes from my joke book. After only about three jokes, Tony's eyelids began to droop. After one or two more jokes, he was flat out asleep. Either he was dead tired or just plain bored with my jokes. I got up to go and didn't want to leave without saying good-bye, yet I hated to wake him.

"I'm leaving, Tony," I said, deciding to wake him. "Happy birthday for tomorrow! I'll be coming back on Friday."

"Okay, Joe," he said faintly. "I apologize for falling asleep. Good-bye."

I glanced at my watch on the way out. It was 12:50."

The Next Day, Visit 25

It was Tony's 85th birthday, and I decided to stop in unannounced and wish him a happy birthday and bring him a small gift. I arrived at 10:15 and brought him a donut with sprinkles of green and white on it, apologizing that it implied Tony was Irish instead of Mediterranean.

"I had a sister who was born on St. Patrick's Day," he said.

He was there all by himself on his birthday, in bed as usual, resting on his back. He looked as though he had been sleeping. I stood near his bed talking to him for about five minutes.

"Bring in a chair and sit down, Joe."

So I did. We talked about a lot of things. I wished him happy birthday, and he seemed real glad I was there.

"I see you have received a bunch of birthday cards, Tony." They were standing on his dresser on the other side of his bed.

"I have such nice friends," he smiled.

"I don't see your lunch anywhere, Tony," I told him. "Did your son forget to fix it for you?"

"My girlfriend, Jane, and her friend, Shirley, are coming over at noon to fix me some lunch and to eat with me. Shirley is in her seventies and is a very attractive woman."

We got to talking about drinking to excess, and Tony confided he had been drunk only twice in his life, both times with Catholic priests.

"Say, Tony, that weekend Gertrude stayed with you while your son went to Wisconsin, did she get fresh with you?" I laughed.

"No, but I wish she had," Tony laughed.

"Did you get out of bed and use your walker to chase her around the apartment?"

"No," he laughed. "But I would have liked to."

"Tony, how about giving me some good advice on how to live to be eighty-five like you."

"I don't think you need any advice, Joe. You seem to be pretty savvy."

He again told me how Guiness Irish dark beer had always been his favorite.

I thought Tony looked especially sleepy today and I wondered if maybe his health was beginning to decline. His mind was very sharp, and he smiled and laughed a lot. He had a small electric heater resting on the cushioned chair by the foot of his bed and asked me to set it on the floor for him, which I did, so the chair would be free for his lady friends. I felt the chair to make sure the heater hadn't got the chair too warm. It hadn't, and I figured it wasn't a fire hazard.

I left at 10:45, feeling good. I had spent 30 minutes with Tony on his birthday. I couldn't get over how sharp he was for being that old. And to think he had all of his teeth, except for one. What a beautiful man he is.

Six Days Later, Visit 26

At about 10 o'clock I called Tony to remind him I would be over at noon to have lunch with him. He said fine, he would be expecting me.

"Hi, Tony. It's me, Joe," I called out, entering the front door of his apartment.

"Hi, Joe," he responded.

I removed some laundry from the living room chair and carried the chair into his bedroom. I saw a partially eaten dish of something or other on his tray and chided Tony for eating his lunch without me. He explained that Robin had already been there and fixed it for him.

He looked very sleepy. I told him I was going to sit down and eat my lunch and talk to him and keep him awake. First I carried his dish, fork, and empty wine glass into the kitchen. I put the dishes in the sink and filled them with water.

"What was that you had for lunch, Tony?"

"Asparagus and boiled eggs. Did you ever have

that?"

"Yes. That's really good."

I sat down and started eating my lunch, a triple-decker peanut butter and strawberry jam sandwich with chopped onions. I smacked my lips and showed Tony the sandwich, and he laughed. I kept talking to him as I ate, keeping him awake. The last thing I ate was a peeled grapefruit, which surprised Tony somewhat, seeing me eat a grapefruit like an orange.

Then I started to read Tony jokes from my joke book. I had to keep waking him. I told him I wanted to stay until 2 o'clock, at which time I had an appointment at the hospice office to get a TB test. He laughed. I succeeded only in keeping him awake until 1:05. I bade him good-bye and left, telling him I would see him next Wednesday.

At the hospice volunteer meeting tonight I met Wendy, who sees Tony on Mondays. I learned that the hospice office is thinking about dropping Tony because he is doing so well. Wendy said she has offered several times to take Tony home with her, but he always declined. I commented how I think Tony wants to die, but his body isn't cooperating. She agreed.

Eight Days Later, Visit 27

I had become a part-time worker with the U.S. Census and didn't arrive at Tony's until 4 o'clock. We chatted a bit and I read him a few jokes, which he seemed to appreciate. His room seemed extra warm, and with Tony's permission, I opened his window a bit. I had some fun pretending that since I was now an official U.S. government

145

worker, I therefore had taken on a lofty importance. Tony laughed when I told him I was now working for Clinton, whom both of us held in low regard. I left at 4:30.

The Next Day, Visit 28

I visited Tony from 12 to 1 o'clock. I ate my lunch, read him some jokes, and opened his window for him again.

Seventeen Days Later, Visit 29

My work with the Census prevented me from visiting Tony until today. At a few minutes after 3 o'clock, I dropped in unannounced. Tony was in bed as usual and seemed glad to see me.

"I'm sorry I haven't been to see you for a few weeks, Tony. It seems that Uncle Sam has been making strong demands on my time." We both laughed.

"I have a very important job," I kidded him, "counting all those Americans out there." We laughed again.

"How are you feeling, Tony?"

"Weaker. I no longer get out of bed to use the commode. My son changes my diaper in the evening and again in the morning. I can't stand up anymore. I'm just too weak."

"Are you still eating good?"

"Yes. For lunch I had a ham and cheese sandwich and my usual small glass of wine."

At about 3:30 a man entered the front door and came into the bedroom. He was big and gregarious, introducing himself to me as Andrew, Tony's son-in-law, married to his daughter Wilma. I felt at ease with his warm and friendly manner. He said he recognized me from our church.

The three of us chatted for half an hour or so. I left at a few minutes after four, telling Tony I would be back on Wednesday, that is if I could break away from the Census work. Otherwise, I told him I would see him as soon as I could make it.

Eleven Days Later, Visit 30

The reason I hadn't seen Tony for 11 days was because my wife fell nine days ago and broke her hip, which changed my life abruptly. Much of my time was suddenly spent in the hospital. For seven days after her surgery I went to the hospital twice a day, and when I brought her home, I found myself in the role of her full-time caregiver.

With my wife's consent, I managed to break away today to visit Tony at 1:30. He was awake and in his usual state of alertness. He said he ate a roast beef sandwich for lunch and drank a small glass of wine his son had left for him.

We chatted for a while; he was very cognitive. He told me again that he no longer gets out of bed, and that his son changes his diaper.

"I need to explain why I haven't been to see you for a while, Tony. My wife fell and broke her hip."

"Oh, no!" Tony interrupted me. "How did it happen?"

"She was wearing socks and snagged a sock on the corner of a cold-air floor ventilator. It

147

threw her off balance and she landed on her right hip. She's had surgery. The doctor fastened the broken bone together with a bolt, four screws, and a plate. The doctor refers to the bolt as a 'pin.' But let me tell you, it's no pin. It's quite a large bolt! She was in the hospital for about a week but is home now. I'm her caregiver. She was resting and I asked her if she would mind if I ran out and visited you for a bit. She said okay."

"Oh, Joe, I'm so sorry to hear that." I could feel the compassion in his voice. "I would like to call her and give her my sympathy."

"You want to call her? Okay. Hey, that would be neat." A silly idea hit me. "I tell you what, Tony. Right after I leave, why don't you call her and ask her if she would like to go dancing with you tonight."

Tony smiled and immediately grasped the humor of it.

"Okay."

I gave him my phone number. I had given my number to him several times already, but gave it to him again, figuring he probably had misplaced it.

He called about an hour after I got home. He told her who he was and, sure enough, he asked her to go dancing with him that evening. I had told my wife I had asked Tony to call her and ask her to go dancing, and she went along with it just great. It was a wonderful phone call. I think it did a lot for both Tony and Dorothy.

I couldn't get over it. A bedridden 85-year-old man dying of colon cancer calling a woman mending with a freshly broken hip, asking her to go dancing! Will wonders ever cease!

Dorothy's breaking her hip forced me to resign as a Census worker so I could become her full-time caregiver.

Five Days Later, Visit 31

At 2:20, once again, with Dorothy's permission, I visited Tony. He was in bed and very drowsy. He said his breathing had become heavy.

"I don't expect to be around much longer, Joe," he said solemnly. I let his statement pass without asking him how much longer he thought he had.

"Would you hand me one of those pain pills," Tony said, pointing to a small vial on his dresser just out of his reach. I handed him one along with a glass of water, and he downed the pill.

"Are you in a lot of pain, Tony?"

"Yes."

"That's so unusual for you. I can't recall your having been in much pain before. Where does it hurt the most?"

"I don't know. Sort of all over."

I removed his lunch dish. His chicken drumstick was only half eaten. His wine glass was empty. Despite his pain and drowsiness, he was very cognitive, warm, and friendly. I left at 3:05 to hurry home to Dorothy.

One Week Later, Visit 32

I dropped in to see Tony at about 1:30 and was met by Florence, whom the family had hired to be Tony's full-time live-in caregiver. She appeared to be of about retirement age.

"Where are you from, Florence?" I asked, mainly because of her accent. I just knew she was going to say she was from Poland.

"Poland."

"Poland? No kidding. Where in Poland?" I had another insight that she was going to say Krakow.

"Krakow."

"Is that right! You are sure doing a good job keeping the apartment neat. I've never seen the apartment looking so clean, and it smells so good in here." I looked around Tony's bedroom. "And Tony's bedroom looks absolutely immaculate!"

I brought along my joke book and read him a couple dozen jokes, which he seemed to enjoy, laughing after most of them and saying, "That's cute."

Although Tony seemed drowsy, he was very cognitive.

"Are you still taking pain medication, Tony?"

"Yes."

He was slurring his words slightly. I wondered if that was because of the pain medicine. I left at about 2:30.

One Week Later, Visit 33

I again dropped in to see Tony at about 1:30 and was met by Florence, his caregiver. The place smelled soapy clean, and Tony's bed and bedroom were impeccably tidy. Tony was again slurring his words but seemed alert.

With his consent, I read him a couple dozen jokes. He again showed his appreciation with laughs, frequently saying, "That's cute."

Florence came in a couple of times to check on things. One time she said she was going outside for some fresh air for five minutes or so. While she was out, Tony asked me to empty his urinating container, which I did.

As I was leaving, I shook hands with Tony and asked him to squeeze my hand as hard as he could. I was amazed at his hand strength. Then I switched hands, shaking hands with him with my left hand and asked him to squeeze again as hard as he could. I was again surprised at his strength.

"Your right hand seems to have a bit more strength, Tony."

"I think you're right, Joe. My right hand is a bit stronger."

Tony thanked me graciously for coming.

I went into the kitchen to say good-bye to Florence, who was standing on a chair wiping down some upper cupboards.

"Be careful, Florence. I wouldn't want you to fall. Otherwise I might have to move in and become the caregiver for both Tony and you," I laughed.

I left at 2:30.

One Week Later, Visit 34

I didn't know it at the time, but today would be the last time I was to see Tony alive. At 2:15, I called out my hello. Florence responded from the

151

kitchen, saying she was having her lunch. I went in to say hello to her.

"Hey, you look like you got your hair done," I told her. "Say, but you look like a movie star now." We both laughed.

I went into Tony's bedroom. He was resting on his back as usual and said he felt sleepy.

"What did you have for lunch, Tony?"

"Some lentil soup and a small glass of wine."

I had my joke book with me, but Tony said he felt too drowsy to listen to them. Instead of sitting down, I elected to remain standing in order to make it easy for Tony to see me.

"Sit down, Joe," Tony told me.

"No. It feels good to stand."

Florence came into the room and she, too, invited me to sit down, but I again declined.

We chatted for a while and, although Tony said he was sleepy, he was very alert and responsive. He said he was again experiencing considerable pain. This time he told me the pain was located in his bowel area. With his colon cancer, I could just imagine the awful extent of his pain.

As I was about to leave, with his permission, I shook his right hand and then his left hand. Each hand grip was firm, with the right hand again exhibiting a bit more strength.

Had I known this was to be the last time I would see Tony alive, I would have told him good-bye. Perhaps I would have prayed with him. I would have stayed longer. I would have thanked him for all the joy he had brought me. I would have told him how fond I had grown of him.

Six Days Later

At about 10 a.m. the hospice office called. My first thought upon recognizing the voice of the caller was that I would be asked to visit another hospice patient. I quickly started conjuring up excuses: I already had a hospice patient, Tony; I still had to do a lot of caregiver chores for my wife while her broken hip mends.

"I just wanted to let you know that Tony died."

Tony died? I was shocked. I just saw him last Wednesday, and he wasn't doing that badly. I was scheduled to see him tomorrow. I felt myself choking up. The hospice office had called me a number of times in the past to tell me my hospice patient had died, but this was the first time I was deeply affected.

"I'm so sorry to hear that. When did he die?" I said, trying to sound matter-of-fact.

"Two days ago. I don't know what time. One of his daughters told me she heard a cough and went into his bedroom to check on him and found him dead."

Tony died only four days after I saw him last.

"You know, I'm genuinely sorry he died. Of course, I knew he was on hospice and dying, but he was so alert. And what a nice guy! I'm really going to miss him. I was supposed to go see him tomorrow."

After I hung up the phone, I told Dorothy about Tony's dying, and found myself sort of breaking down. This was the first hospice patient death that deeply moved me. No wonder. I had been visiting Tony once or twice a week for six months!

"I'm going to miss him," I told Dorothy. I felt my eyes growing foggy with tears. "I really did enjoy visiting with him. What a nice man!"

The hospice office called back a few minutes later to ask if I could spend five hours next Thursday visiting a new hospice patient. I told her I couldn't because Dorothy had two doctor appointments that day. I told once again how deeply Tony's death affected me, because I had really got to know him.

I checked today's newspaper and found Tony's death notice. His wake was indeed going to be in the funeral home so readily visible out the kitchen window of his apartment! His wake and funeral were scheduled for tomorrow. I decided to attend both. After all, Tony was special.

The Next Day

I headed for the funeral home just as though I were going to Tony's apartment. Seeing Tony's apartment building on my right, I turned left into the funeral home parking lot. I got out of my car and glanced over my shoulder at Tony's kitchen window. I remembered asking Tony if his body would be taken to this funeral home, and I recalled his answer: "I don't know, and I don't care. I'll let them surprise me." I could still see his smile when he said that. Then I headed for the funeral home entrance. I looked at my watch. It was 9:30.

I went into the big parlor where Tony's body was lying in state and was greeted by his daughter Kay. I felt myself blush as she corrected me. I had mistakenly called her Wilma, her sister's name. While we were talking, Wilma came up and joined us. Then Tony's son approached. All three were prolific in praising me for all the good work I did in visiting Tony. I was quick to tell them my thoughts about their father, what a great man I thought he was, and how in visiting hospice patients, how I receive so much more than I give.

I was introduced to a man who joined us, Calhoun, who said he has known Tony for years. Calhoun was tall, handsome, and looked very Irish. He told how he remembered Tony stopping at his home frequently and patiently showing him how to do various tasks.

I found myself enjoying talking with Calhoun, not noticing that Kay, Wilma, and Tony Jr. had drifted off. He was prolific in his praise for me and for other hospice volunteers. I told him also how I gain so much more than I give when I visit a hospice patient.

Calhoun was so friendly. I could have talked with him much longer. But I broke away and went to kneel down in front of the casket to look at Tony. He was impeccably dressed for his great encounter with the next life. Pinstripe suit and matching tie. His mustache was freshly trimmed. I silently talked to him. How happy I am for you, Tony, that you are finally at peace, no longer suffering, no longer bound to that bed. How sad I felt when I was told of your death. I really and truly choked up. I grew terribly fond of you, Tony.

I think you were the nicest man I ever met. Now you know all about the afterlife, whether anything is there. I hope you found an all-loving God, and I hope this God rewarded you with a cozy spot in his heaven.

Exiting the funeral home I picked up a remembrance card from the desk. On one side was printed the Prayer of St. Francis:

"Make me an instrument of Your peace;
Where there is hatred, let me sow love;
Where there is injury, pardon;
Where there is doubt, faith;
Where there is despair, hope;
Where there is darkness, light;
And where there is sadness, joy.
Grant that I may not so much seek to be consoled
as to console;
To be understood as to understand;
To be loved as to love;
For it is in pardoning that we are pardoned,
And it is in dying that we are born to eternal life."

Walking to my car, I again looked at the kitchen window on the second floor of Tony's apartment. I thought about how the door to the apartment was always unlocked. I wondered if Tony Jr. would now start locking the door. I wondered further if Tony Jr. would continue living there. I looked at my watch. It was only 10:15. The funeral mass wouldn't begin until 11:30. I decided to go home for a while and then set out for the mass.

I parked in front of the church at 11 o'clock. Why was I arriving half an hour early? As I walked past the rectory, I noticed a man leaving. He wasn't dressed like a priest, but I thought maybe he could be a priest. He had on a sport shirt and dark pants and was heading for the church.

I went inside the church vestibule and saw a man and woman perhaps my age, probably husband and wife. I started chatting with them, and then the man from the rectory joined us. When the couple called him "Father," it was obvious that he was a priest. I asked if he were the musician to play for the funeral. He replied that, yes, he was.

"At my church we have an all-volunteer choir that sings at funerals. Does your church have such a choir for funerals?"

"No," the priest replied.

"Are you going to play the organ and sing for the funeral?" I asked him.

"Yes."

The priest turned and headed toward the aisle on the east side of the church. Our youngest daughter was married in this church, and I figured he was heading for the organ, located on that side of the church about a third of the way from the altar. I decided to sit near the organ to observe the priest. I also had another motive. I intended to ask him if I could sing with him during the mass. Having sung with our funeral choir many times, I knew the favorite funeral hymns well. I was confident I could do a good job with him and, perhaps, enhance the music program. Wouldn't Tony be proud?

I took a seat across the aisle from the organ

and watched as the priest prepared his music. A microphone attached to a rod was positioned near his mouth for him to sing into as he played. I thought maybe I could stand near him and sing with him.

I waited for a few minutes and then asked him, "Father, I know the funeral hymns, having sung them many times in our funeral choir. Could I join you in singing?" I thought sure he would say yes and welcome me to stand near him and sing with him. I was certain also that Tony would like it if I sang with the priest.

"No," he said abruptly and firmly and began to play one of the hymns, "Eagle's Wings," one of my favorites.

I was miffed. I felt like getting up and leaving, or at least moving away from the priest and sitting somewhere else. But I remained where I was.

Soon the casket was wheeled up the center aisle to a position in front of the altar, and family members positioned themselves in the front pew on the left.

I studied the priest as he played the organ and sang. He did very well. I thought his voice was pleasant. Not outstanding, but adequate. I kept thinking of what Tony had told me during one of my visits. "All priests are queers (homosexuals)." I studied the priest celebrant and the one playing the organ and singing. Were they? I had no idea.

When I went to communion, I walked past Tony, Wilma, and Kay, and looked straight ahead, avoided their eyes. I didn't want them to think I was attending just for show.

I wanted to linger around after mass and compliment the priest organist-singer, but got caught up in the exiting procedure. Outside the church I went to my car and thought I was trapped in the funeral procession. A man came by and asked if I was going to the cemetery, and I said no. I had decided to wait until the funeral procession left, but then a car went past me heading out, and I followed. I was home about 10 minutes later.

I told Dorothy about the priest musician-singer and how he didn't want me to join him. Dorothy took the side of the priest, which I knew she would, saying I had a lot of gall asking if I could join him. I told her how he had said no instantly. "How was he to know I didn't have a voice like Placido Domingo? I think the priest was filled with pride and wanted all the glory as the sole performer."

Later, reflecting on the whole thing, I sort of marveled at my boldness in volunteering to sing with the priest. It really wasn't like me to do that. What had got into me?

About a Month Later

I received a thank-you card from Tony's son, which read as follows:

"To know you are with us
in our time of sorrow.
Sharing our prayers,
today and tomorrow.
God gives us comfort
in the form of family and friends

May His peace be with you,
His love never ends.
By the family of"
(signed) Tony Jr.

Shawn

Thursday

The hospice office called to give me a new patient: Shawn, 74, in real bad shape with emphysema and heart failure, a patient in a home care center. His wife, Eileen, needs daily rides to see her husband. I called Eileen, and she said she had a ride on Friday but would need a ride one day next week.

Monday

On Monday Eileen called and asked me to give her a ride on Wednesday. We agreed I would pick her up at her home at 1:30.

Wednesday

Her house was easy to find. I drove slowly past, failing to see her house number. I saw a woman sitting on the porch and figured it was she. I turned around at the end of the block and came back, and she waved, knowing it would be me. I pulled into her driveway, and she went in the house briefly and came back out and got in the car. It was about 1:25.

I introduced myself and showed her my hospice badge to prove I was "official." On the way to the home care center, we talked about odds and ends. She said she and Shawn had been married for 17 years, that it was her second marriage. She has children by her first marriage, and Shawn, two children by his first marriage.

Eileen said Shawn had heart bypass surgery five years ago and has had a number of heart attacks since. He had been hospitalized for three weeks and was finally put on hospice and has been in the home care center for a week.

When we came to the facility, we parked and went in the front door. She stopped at the office and greeted a woman inside, asking how her Shawn was doing. An attractive woman named Maggie replied that he was doing well. I asked Maggie if she were the boss, and she said, no, she was the assistant manager, that the manager was away on his honeymoon. We went around the corner to our left and walked toward the end of the corridor and turned left into room 104. Her husband was in the bed by the window; the other bed was empty, its occupant had gone to the sitting room.

Shawn appeared to be in very bad shape. He was lying on his back, covered to his chest with a sheet and white blanket. His facial skin coloring was a whitish pink. His hair, white with some thinning, needed brushing. His eyes were brown. He was wearing a clear-plastic oxygen mask over his nose and mouth.

Eileen greeted him with a kiss and introduced me. He held out his hand for me to shake. I grasped it and squeezed it with both hands, telling him how glad I was to meet him.

During most of the time I was there, Shawn kept using his right hand and forefinger to nudge Eileen and indicate he wanted something. She would have to guess at what he wanted, because he wasn't able to speak. She would ask him something like, "Do you want water?" He would shake his head negative. "Do you want Coke?" Negative shake. "Do you want your milk shake?" Affirmative shake. He didn't let her alone the whole time she was there, indicating some want: milk shake, water, Coke, pain medicine, scratch his leg, move his leg, call the nurse, etc. Eileen stood by his bed on Shawn's right, and I was on his left.

I made some conversation with him. I got sort of a game going with him trying to guess his birth date by the process of elimination. He indicated he was 72, although I knew he was actually 74. I then set out to guess his weight (200 pounds), also by the process of elimination. I tried to guess where in Tennessee one of his children lived, but Shawn, no matter what city I named, shook his head negatively. I finally gave up; I couldn't think of any more cities to name.

At one point Eileen left the room for about 10 minutes to summon the nurse and left me alone with Shawn. During this time Shawn kept indicating to me he wanted something.

Eileen had initially rung for the nurse, but after about 15 minutes a black guy arrived, apologizing for not getting there sooner. He walked into the room very slowly, shaking his head and groaning how tired he was because he was having to work two floors. I introduced myself to him, put my hand out to shake his, and asked him his name. "J.R." he said, shaking my hand warmly and smiling. This bit of attention seemed to energize him. He complimented me for my warm grip.

A very pretty young lady came into the room and identified herself as Candy, the social worker for the place, and said she had brought Shawn a milk shake and had given it to him to drink, and that he had drunk most of it. She said she would bring him a milk shake daily, and Eileen gave her a $5 bill to cover the cost.

Shawn's roommate patient came into the room and identified himself as Don. He had what appeared to be ice cream stains on his T-shirt and changed it. I marveled that he had all his belongings in a small locker by his bed. He didn't have any teeth and was chomping his jaw. He seemed real friendly.

A woman, probably 85 or so, sitting in a wheelchair, wheeled herself to Shawn's side and held his hand. She kept muttering something unintelligible, and I asked Eileen what she was saying. She said she was praying. The lady stayed about 10 minutes and left.

Eileen told me that Shawn is related to a past mayor of a certain large city. She said Shawn loves Italian cooking, especially pasta, and hates German and Irish cooking. She asked him if he wanted her to bring him some pasta, and he nodded affirmatively. I asked her what kind of pasta he likes, and she said any kind, as long as it has a red sauce on it.

At 3:20 I began to think we should be leaving or else I would be caught in heavy traffic driving home. I suggested that I could go home and, if she wanted to stay, I could come back and get her at about 6 o'clock. At first she said that would be fine, then changed her mind abruptly and decided to go with me.

I shook Shawn's hand warmly and told him how glad I was to meet him.

I got home by 4:05, very sleepy, and stretched out and closed my eyes for about 30 minutes.

I thought about my experience. Shawn is in very bad shape. Eileen said she keeps praying for the Lord to take him. He is really suffering. All he can move is his head back and forth, and his hands and arms. He has a terrible-sounding cough, as though his lungs contain some liquid. Eileen said he has stopped eating and is having trouble swallowing. But every time she gave him a drink of water, Coke, or milk shake, he seemed to swallow nicely.

Shawn had some dark blotches on his hands and arms, probably from being stuck with needles so many times. He no longer has any needles in him. He wears diapers. J.R. said he had changed Shawn shortly before we arrived.

I remember telling Shawn I thought he looked like he would make a good priest. Eileen laughed and said Shawn was no priest. She didn't elaborate.

Judging from Shawn's state of health, I figured he would be dying at any time, that he certainly wouldn't make it more than a few days.

Just as Eileen got out of my car, she deposited a $5 bill on the passenger seat. "This is for gas," she said.

"You don't have to give me gas money," I replied. But she closed the door and headed for her front door.

Wednesday

The hospice office called to tell me Shawn had died Tuesday afternoon. For the next few days I searched the newspaper for his obituary notice, but never found it. A week or so later I mailed the $5 bill back to Eileen. I thanked her for the privilege of driving her one time to see her husband, and for the joy of getting to meet and talk to him. About a week later I received a thank-you card from her. It read, "An extra special thank you for everything! Your thoughtfulness is warmly appreciated!"

Bert

Thursday

The hospice office called and assigned me a new patient: Bert, 80, lung cancer, a stroke reduced the use of his right arm. She asked me to sit with him on Monday, Wednesday, and Friday from 2 until about 6:30 while his wife, Eleanor, goes in for dialysis. Their house is up for sale, and they hope to move by the end of next month. He is on oxygen and can't be left alone. I accepted the assignment, and immediately called Eleanor to assure her I could be there. She said I needed to arrive by 2:10 so she could reach the hospital by 2:30 for her dialysis.

Monday, Visit 1

At about 1 o'clock I called Eleanor to verify their house location. She said I could park in their driveway. I arrived at the residence at 1:57. They had a double driveway but only a single-car garage. An older car was parked on the left side of the driveway.

It's funny, but I had driven past this attractive brick ranch home a million times without ever noticing it. Carrying my briefcase and Thermos, I rang the doorbell, and moments later I was introducing myself to Eleanor, showing her my hospice badge to assure her I was "official." I was struck by her stately beauty. She was my height, had an erect posture, held her head high, and

167

was soft-spoken.

She led me through a living room to a large family room at the back of the house. I set my briefcase and Thermos on a table on the west side of the room. Her husband, Bert, was lying on his back in a hospital bed along the east wall of the room and had an oxygen mask on his face. The head of his bed was raised slightly so he could watch a large TV about 10 feet in front and slightly to the left of him. The TV was playing rather loudly.

She introduced me to him, and we shook hands without his sitting up. I pressed his hand firmly with both of my hands and told him how glad I was to meet him.

Eleanor was preparing to leave and told me her dialysis takes three hours, "but longer by the time they stop the bleeding." She said she would likely be back at about 6:30. I told her not to hurry, that I was retired and had nowhere special to go. I felt sorry for her, having to go in for dialysis. In fact, I felt sorry for both of them: Bert, dying with lung cancer and with a recent stroke, and Eleanor, with failing kidneys.

She said she was pretty certain they had sold their house, and they were beginning to make plans to move to a condo.

She asked me to call the oxygen-supply company after 3 o'clock "if they haven't come by then," and tell them Bert's oxygen tanks need to be recharged.

"I brought along my joke book. It's full of jokes that poke fun at us older folks," I smiled. "A lot of them are really funny. Maybe after while I'll read some to Bert, that is, if he wants me to."

Eleanor smiled, and Bert stared at the TV.

"Bert can go to the bathroom all right, but you may have to help him," she said. And then she was gone. I found myself standing by Bert's bed looking down at him. He seemed to be concentrating on the TV program, an old Bonanza rerun.

"So you're watching Bonanza, eh, Bert?" I said cheerfully.

"Yeah," he said matter-of-factly.

I saw a chair nearby and pulled it up close to Bert's bed and sat down. The chair was equipped with caster wheels.

"Mind if I sit here and watch the program with you?"

"No, go right ahead," he said, continuing to watch TV.

I looked at Bert. He had a short haircut, wore glasses, and had on dark blue pajamas. My eyes drifted from his clear-plastic oxygen mask down along a plastic tube, which was attached to three oxygen tanks about 10 feet away.

Then I noticed that Bert was asleep. I quietly pushed the chair back to the table where my briefcase and Thermos were, and sat down. I got up and found the remote control and lowered the TV volume somewhat. I opened my briefcase and took out a book to read. I suddenly found myself getting interested in the Bonanza program.

Minutes later I noticed Bert stirring, and I went to his side.

"Is there anything I can do for you, Bert?"

"No."

"Do you need to go to the bathroom?"

"No, not yet."

"Okay, I'm sitting over there by that table. Holler if you want anything. Okay?"

"Okay."

I began to study the decor in the room. The north wall, where the TV was located, had some cupboards and an alcove with yellow and green stained-glass windows. The east wall had cream-colored brick, two windows, and two book shelves below the windows. The west wall was mostly windows, looking out on the back yard, with two chairs, lamp, a round table and four chairs, each chair on casters. The south wall had windows that looked out on a roofed patio.

Their carpet was a light brown, and I thought it was identical to the carpeting Dorothy and I have in our home.

Then I noticed that Bert was barefoot, that his oxygen mask had a little bag under it, and that Bert's breathing seemed to be rather heavy.

At 2:45 Bert asked me to help him to the bathroom. Well, this ought to be interesting.

"Can I help you get up?"

"No, I can get up by myself."

"Okay."

When he stood up, he removed his oxygen mask, leaving it on his bed.

"Just sort of hold my arm in case I should need help," he said. He barked out his request in the form of a command, not unlike that of an Army drill sergeant. He apparently was used to bossing people around. Perhaps he had been a manager somewhere.

After we went just a few feet, I felt Bert easing off to the right, and he shouted, "Grab me! I'm going to fall."

I quickly grasped his left arm with both hands and pulled him back to me.

"Hey, Bert. You tried to get away from me there, didn't you?" I laughed.

"Yeah."

"Good thing I was hanging on to you," I laughed again. But I could feel my heart pounding. It was a good thing indeed I had had a firm grip on his arm, or he really would have fallen and could have been badly injured.

In the bathroom he said he couldn't use his hands very well, and he asked me to raise the lid of the toilet for him so he could sit down.

"You don't go standing up?"

"No. I have to sit down."

I raised the top lid for him.

"Okay, Bert."

"Now, would you pull down my pajamas for me. With my stroke, it's hard for me to do."

"Sure, no problem."

I felt under his pajama top for the top of his pajama pants and pulled them down to near his knees.

"Thanks. That's fine. Now you can go out and close the door. I'll call you when I'm done."

"Okay."

I did as he said, going out and closing the door. Minutes later he called and said he was done. I entered the bathroom and Bert was still sitting on the toilet.

"Help me get up."

"Okay."

I reached under his left arm and pulled him to a standing position.

"Now pull up my pajamas."

"Okay."

Then I held his arm firmly as he walked slowly back to his bed. He sat down on the bed, and I put the oxygen mask on him, and he leaned back, resting his head on his pillow.

"What else can I do for you, Bert?"

"Let's hear a couple of those jokes," he said.

"How about if we wait until Bonanza is over," I suggested. I had been watching it and wanted to see how it ended. "Little Joe" had been in an Army stockade and was to be shot for a crime he didn't commit. I just had to see the ending and watch his dad and brother come to his rescue, which they did, just as Army sharpshooters were about to fire their rifles at him.

"Okay, Bert, I'm ready to read you some jokes."

I pulled up my chair to the side of his bed. Opening the book at random, I started to read. He showed a great sense of humor, laughing at each joke, which poked fun at oldsters. After half a dozen or so jokes, Bert's eyes shut and he started breathing heavily. He was fast asleep. I moved the chair back to the table and put away the joke book.

Bert began tossing and turning restlessly, and

I went to his side to see if his eyes were open. They were.

"You woke up, Bert. I see your oxygen mask has slipped down. Let me adjust it for you." The mask had slipped downward several inches. I moved the mask back into place to cover his nose and mouth and tucked the elastic support strings behind his head.

"There, Bert. How's that? That mask seems to want to keep slipping down on you."

"Yeah. Something's wrong with the design. It doesn't want to stay in place."

I stood by his bed and continued chatting with him. By standing, I could make better eye contact with him than by sitting next to his bed. Here are some of the things we talked about:

- Bert said he designed and built the family room, which was a large addition to the house.
- Bert and Eleanor had lived in this house for 51 years.
- They have four children, 10 grandchildren, and 10 great-grandchildren.
- Bert used to design store interiors.
- He said his wife tends to get preoccupied with her dialysis and forgets to leave him a snack.
- He showed me a hat given to him by one of his sons. The hat contained a number of comical messages.
- He complained about the fee he and his wife would have to pay to the real estate agent for selling their house, "about

$19,000." He said the selling fee was 6%.

- Their house was built in 1947, two years before they moved into it. It is all brick, and has a half basement.
- Bert built the family room addition and the enclosed patio 30 years ago.
- Bert said that regarding his stroke, "the doctor got it wrong. It wasn't so much my right hand that was affected, but both hands." He said he can't pick up things anymore. He demonstrated this to me. His hands could go to an object but could not grasp it. He couldn't even adjust his oxygen mask. He said he had the stroke about six weeks ago. Bert said he had just recently turned 80.

At 3:30 I remembered that Eleanor had told me to call the oxygen company if they hadn't come by 3 o'clock, because Bert's supply of oxygen was low. I found the number on one of the three oxygen tanks and was told by the dispatcher that a truck was on the way.

Meanwhile, Bert said he was feeling strange and asked me to get his medicine for him. Recalling a recent reminder to me that hospice volunteers are not allowed to administer medicine, I proceeded with caution. Bert had me bring two small boxes of medicine to him and read him the names. He couldn't remember the name of the medicine he wanted but said he would remember it if he heard it. I read him the names of each medicine container three times. All the while Bert was cussing and swearing pretty good. Not at me, but simply because the medicine wasn't being found. Finally I got the bright idea to call hospice. The hospice nurse checked Bert's records and said he was taking something called Vicodin. I told her he had no medicine by that name. She said maybe he had the generic version, "hydrocodone." I told her that, yes, he had a medicine by that name. She said that was it, to give him two of those pills. She said Bert had a liquid medicine called Roxanol, for severe pain, but not to give him that. I got the hydrocodone container and showed Bert one of the pills.

"That's it," he said.

Since he was unable to grasp things due to his stroke, I put a pill in his mouth, gave him a sip of water, and repeated this. But Bert still wasn't satisfied.

"Call my doctor and ask if there's anything else I should take," he ordered. He said the doctor's phone number was in a little book that Eleanor kept near the phone in the kitchen. I found the book and the number for his doctor. Minutes later I was actually speaking to the doctor. I told him I had just given Bert two Vicodin pills. He said not to give him anything else, that those two pills ought to ease his anxiety. He told me to make sure Bert wears his oxygen mask at all times. He used a big word to describe Bert's condition, indicating his blood supply is oxygen-starved.

I told Bert what the doctor said, and this seemed to soothe him.

Then the oxygen truck came. Two black guys, Harry, and Doc, his helper-in-training, recharged the three tanks. They said to tell Eleanor they have ordered a portable oxygen tank for Bert but it hadn't come in yet. Bert wanted the portable tank so he could attend a wedding. Bert's three tanks run out every three days; he uses 5 liters per minute from each tank.

A few minutes after the oxygen truck left, I noticed a fog-like substance cascading down the sides of a tank. Thinking that it must be leaking oxygen, I called the oxygen company, and a voice told me not to be concerned, that this often happens after oxygen tanks are recharged, that it should stop after 30 minutes or so. And, indeed, it stopped after about that much time.

Because of what the doctor told me, I now started checking Bert's oxygen mask frequently to make sure it was where it was supposed to be. The mask kept slipping down on his face. I unbuttoned the top button on his pajama top and tucked the oxygen tube between the top two buttons to help prevent him from accidentally pulling the mask down. After a while I saw that this wasn't working and restored the tube to where it was.

At 5 o'clock Bert said he "had to pee" and he wanted to use the portable commode near his bed. He had me pull his pajama bottoms down, and I assisted him to sit on the commode. He said he "sits to pee." I asked him if he had ever been "reamed out." He said he had had the operation a few years earlier, "but the doctor botched it."

When he finished, I helped him up and pulled up his pajamas. Then I emptied the commode bucket and rinsed it out.

I asked Bert what his real first name was.

"My full name is Bertrand David," he replied.

"How did you ever get a name like Bertrand? Was that your mother's maiden name?"

"No," Bert laughed. "You won't believe this, but my dad named me for a tramp who lived along the Mississippi River."

"What? You got to be kidding!"

"It's true. And he gave me the middle name of 'Dee.' But I couldn't stand that and changed it to David. But everyone calls me 'Bert.'"

"That's really interesting."

"I have one brother and three sisters."

"Hey, Bert. There's a fly on the window. Is there a flyswatter some place?"

"Yeah, there's one in the kitchen."

I went into the kitchen and looked around but couldn't find one. I found a magazine and rolled it up and returned to the window. The fly had moved to a part of the window immediately behind some drapes. I quickly pushed the drapes against the fly, dispatching it to insect heaven.

"I got it, Bert. I didn't even need a swatter," I bragged.

"Good job," he laughed.

I got to studying the top of Bert's left hand.

"Your hand looks bruised, Bert. What happened to it?"

"That was from when I was in the hospital when I had my stroke. They stuck a lot of needles in that hand."

I began to look at his feet. He had enormous big toes. But I thought it would have been inappropriate to tell him that.

I idly glanced at the wall on the other side of

his bed. I counted six framed pictures, probably 9 by 12 inches; two framed collage-type pictures, likely about 20 by 24 inches; a round artistic arrangement with a dried flower, probably 3 feet in diameter; a large star-like clock with four long points and four short points. The clock's points were black, and it had gold hands, with no numbers.

I thought it seemed stuffy in the room, and, with Bert's permission, I turned off the air conditioner and opened some windows in the family room. Ah, I felt better already!

In talking with Bert, I learned that Wednesday would be Eleanor's birthday. I made a mental note to wish her a happy birthday upon my arrival Wednesday.

At about 5:15 I pulled up a chair alongside Bert's bed, and we started chatting. I kept adjusting his mask, which kept slipping down from his nose and mouth. "The doctor told me it was vitally important for you to keep that mask on and breathe in oxygen," I told him.

Something prompted me to test the strength in each of Bert's hands. I grasped his right hand in my right hand, as though we were going to shake hands, and asked him to squeeze as hard as he could. His strength surprised me; his grip was quite firm. I did the same thing with his left hand. It, too, had considerable strength.

"Bert, I'm surprised that you have such strength in your hands, what with your stroke."

Bert expressed surprise, too, especially since he was unable to use his fingers to pick up anything. I noticed that the fingers on his right hand turned in somewhat toward his palm, and that in order to grip his hand, I had to pull back his fingers somewhat.

"What's that big tree behind your house, Bert?" I figured it was a Siberian elm, but wanted to hear what Bert thought it was.

"It's a Chinese elm."

"A Chinese elm? Interesting. It sure is big. Has it ever been struck by lighting?"

"No. But a big limb fell off during a storm and broke through the roof over the patio. It cost $12,000 to repair the roof."

"It cost $12,000?"

"Yeah. That roof is made with two-inch-thick redwood."

"Oh, no wonder." I went to the window to study the roof and admired the redwood framing.

I looked back at the tree and estimated its age at somewhere around 75 years.

"So you say you're a designer. Tell me about something you designed."

He laughed. "I designed a lot of things, especially stores. One that comes to mind is a gift shop at a hospital."

"And, you say you're not an architect?"

"No. I almost am, though. I could probably hold my own against a lot of architects."

Thinking for a moment about his lung cancer, I felt compelled to ask him, "Did you smoke cigarettes for a long time?"

"Yeah, for forty years."

"At what age did you start and quit?"

"I didn't start until I was forty, and I quit just

recently, when I had my stroke and was hospitalized. That was when they diagnosed me with inoperable lung cancer and put me on hospice."

"How long ago was this?"

"I had my stroke six weeks ago."

"And, before the stroke, you apparently were in good health?"

"Yes."

"Your breathing was good? And you cut the grass? And you were quite active?"

"Yes."

"You don't seem to have a cough."

"No. No cough."

"Do you have pain from the lung cancer?"

"No."

I asked Bert which daughter was in the collage.

"That's Rebecca."

"Rebecca is so very pretty! And so is your other daughter, Amanda. The pictures show that Amanda seems to have almost a classic beauty. Your daughters are so pretty!"

"Thank-you."

"Who is in the picture at the far right?"

"That's my brother and his wife."

"Your wife looks as though she may be somewhat younger than you, Bert."

"She's seven years younger. She's seventy-three."

"You're both Leos?"

"No. Just me. I don't know what Eleanor is.

She's that sign that comes after Leo."

After I readjusted Bert's oxygen mask for the umtieth time, I thought maybe if I taped the mask to his face it wouldn't slip off. I asked Bert if he had any duct tape. He said there was a roll on his work bench in the basement. With his permission I went down to the basement and brought up the tape. Minutes later I had ripped off two small pieces and taped the sides of his mask to the sides of his face and to his forehead.

"There, Bert. By gosh, I think that might do the trick. Does the tape bother you? Does it feel uncomfortable?"

"No, it feels fine."

"How does it feel to be put on hospice, Bert? Is it scary?"

"No. I knew that sooner or later something like this was coming."

"As I get older, I find I'm no longer afraid to die," I told him, looking for his reaction.

"I'm the same way. I used to be afraid to die. But now that I'm old, I no longer fear it."

"Do you believe in an afterlife?"

"Yes."

"What religion are you, Bert?"

"Christian."

"When they put you on hospice, did they give you an expected time to live?"

"No."

I knew I was on dangerous ground, that I would have to be careful in what I was about to say.

"I think most people when they are put on

181

hospice are usually given six months or less to live." I added quickly, "Don't quote me on that. Any kind of a prediction on remaining lifespan needs to come from your doctor."

I paused and then asked, "How long have you lived in this house, Bert?"

"We bought the house in 1949 and have lived here for fifty-one years. We raised four children in this house."

"You had two boys and two girls. I suppose you had two boys sleeping in one bedroom, and two girls in a bedroom?"

"Yeah."

"You have only one bathroom?"

"No, a bath and a half. I put a toilet and sink in the basement."

"Bert, I notice there's a car next to mine in your driveway. Is that your car?"

"Yes."

"What kind of car is it?"

"It's a 1983 Chevrolet Caprice."

"A 1983? Wow!"

"I want to sell it."

"Maybe you could give it to one of your grandchildren. Did you serve in the military in World War II?"

"No. When I went to enlist, I was rejected because they told me my heart was on my right side instead of on my left."

"Is that right? But, here you are eighty years old. Did that ever bother you?"

"No," he laughed. "My heart has always

worked just fine."

"That's really tough that Eleanor has to go in for dialysis," I said.

"Yeah. She also has diabetes."

"Oh, no!" I wasn't sure why I reacted with such surprise. Probably because I had heard that diabetes complicates most diseases.

"It's amazing how much water they get out of her during that dialysis," he said.

"How's your appetite, Bert? Do you eat good?"

"Yeah."

"What did you have for breakfast?"

"A bowl of cereal, two pieces of jam toast, and a glass of apple juice."

"Hey, that's a good-sized breakfast."

"What is your normal height and weight, Bert?"

"I'm an even six feet and used to weigh a hundred ninety-four."

"Wow! You're a big guy!"

"I think I lost some of that weight, though, since I had my stroke."

"Bert, you look good. You have a good healthy coloring, and your mind is sharp!"

"Thanks. Yeah, I feel good, except, of course, for the stroke. I can't use my fingers very well."

"What color eyes do you have, Bert?"

"Brown."

It was 6:45 when Eleanor returned. I thought she looked a bit queasy from her dialysis.

"Hi, Eleanor. Do you feel all right?" I asked.

"Yes. I feel fine."

I didn't see her car in the driveway and asked her, "Where did you park?"

"Across the street in that parking lot. That place of business is up for sale."

"You parked over there?" I felt bad. She had moved her car to the lot across the street so I could park in her driveway. "You didn't have to do that. When I come Wednesday, I'll park across the street so you won't have to move your car."

"All right."

I told her how I had called the hospice nurse to find out about Bert's medicine. I showed her the container of hydrocodone and how I had penciled the word "Vicodin" on it's label. I told her also how at Bert's urging, I had called his doctor, and what the doctor had told me to do, not to give him any more medicine, and to make sure he was getting his oxygen.

"Bert said he's really getting hungry. He told me you were going to fix him a big steak when you got home," I laughed. She wasn't sure I was joking, so I added, "I was just kidding. He didn't really say that."

I told her how I had taped Bert's oxygen mask to his face because it kept slipping off. "It doesn't look very sightly, but it seems to be holding the mask in place. And Bert said he doesn't mind the tape," I smiled.

As I was leaving, I added, "I'll be happy to come back and sit with Bert on Wednesday and Friday. I'll see you at two o'clock on Wednesday."

She thanked me, and I was on my way home. Driving home, I reflected on my visit with Bert. I had helped him go to the bathroom three times and helped him once to his portable commode. I had to pull down his pajama bottoms and raise them for him each time.

After I got home, I made a mental note to bring some Band-Aids with me on Wednesday to use to tape Bert's oxygen mask to his face, because the duct tape is so unsightly.

Wednesday, Visit 2

At a few minutes before 2 o'clock, I parked in the vacant lot across the street so Eleanor wouldn't have to move her car. I glanced over at the house, and a car backed out to permit another car to back out and leave, and then the first car pulled back into the driveway. I crossed the street and met the driver as he exited his car and headed for the front door.

"Hi. My name is Joe, and I'm a hospice volunteer, coming to sit with Bert while Eleanor goes in for her dialysis," I said cheerily.

The man was about my height and was nice looking and precisely groomed. I thought he might be Bert's doctor.

"Hi. I'm Pastor Robert. I'm here to give communion to Bert. I just had to move my car so the nurse could leave. I had her car blocked in the driveway."

"Hi, Pastor Robert." I knew from the title he gave himself that he couldn't be a Catholic priest. I suspected he was Anglican. "What church are you pastor of?" I thought this was a bit more subtle than asking him his religion.

"St. Mary Anglican Church." I was right.

"Oh. Is that located right across from the park?"

"Yes. That's it."

We went inside and were greeted by Eleanor.

"I used to work with a fellow who graduated from the St. Mary Anglican Grammar School."

"Is that right?"

We went into the family room, and I greeted Bert. Pastor Robert sat down and continued with his services, which he had interrupted to move his car. Seconds later we were all reciting the Our Father. As Pastor Robert was making his exit, he commented that Bert's lavender pajamas matched Eleanor's outfit. I mentally thanked him for his observation. I wouldn't have noticed it. It was true; they did match!

Before leaving home to sit with Bert, I had researched the difference between a Chinese elm and a Siberian elm. Bert had told me the giant tree close to the back of his house was a Chinese elm. I thought it to be a Siberian elm, but then realized I didn't know the difference between the two. I learned that the Chinese elm (Ulmus parvifolio) is also called the lacebark elm, and has bark that flakes off in small chips; it also flowers and bears seeds in the fall rather than in the spring. The Siberian elm (Ulmus pumila) flowers and produces an abundant wind-borne seed in the spring. It has become a weed in landscapes and waste ground.

"Does your elm flower and seed in the spring or fall?" I asked Eleanor.

"The spring," she replied readily.

"Then, it's a Siberian elm instead of a Chinese

elm," I smiled, explaining to her and Bert that I had researched the subject. I didn't want to tell them it was a "weed" tree. Bert said they had planted the tree some 30 years ago. I was surprised. Judging from the immense trunk, I had guessed it was perhaps 75 years old. So ended the saga of their huge elm tree, which had dropped a limb during a storm, crushing the expensive redwood roof over their patio.

Overnight I had thought about whether or not I wanted to make a commitment to continue sitting for Bert while Eleanor went for dialysis. I had told Barbara and Eleanor I would do it Monday, Wednesday, and Friday of this week, and then would make a decision. But I had already made up my mind.

"Eleanor, I've decided to continue sitting with Bert after this week."

She thanked me. There, I made the commitment, and I was glad. I liked Bert, and I liked Eleanor. I liked sitting with Bert, because it made me feel needed, staying with him while his wife went to a hospital for dialysis. With Bert's inability to use his hands fully, he really needed help.

"Do you feel anything when you are undergoing dialysis?" I asked her.

"No, not a thing. I usually doze off or try to read."

"And, you don't feel a thing?"

"I feel them inserting the needle. That is usually quite painful. But after that, I don't feel anything."

I had figured that maybe a person undergoing

dialysis would feel perhaps light-headed or something like that.

"I parked across the street so you won't have to move your car," I told her.

She thanked me, and then reminded me to give Bert at 3:15 two pills she had set out on his tray. Then she was gone.

Right after she left I could have kicked myself. I had forgot to wish her happy birthday. Bert had told me on Monday today would be her 73rd birthday! I had made a mental note to congratulate her. Oh, well, I'll try to remember when she comes back from dialysis.

"Bert, I see the duct tape is no longer on your oxygen mask."

"It didn't stick very good, so we took it off."

"It was real unsightly, too," I laughed. "But guess what. I've brought along some Band-Aids to use to tape the mask to your face. This won't be nearly as unsightly as the duct tape. Would you mind if I use them?"

"No, go right ahead."

I proceeded to put a Band-Aid on each side of his mask, taping them to his jaws, and another Band-Air to the top of his mask, taping it to his forehead.

"There, Bert! Now you're all set. Now that darn mask isn't going to slip off."

"Okay," Bert laughed.

I sat by his bed and we started to chat.

"Do you want to watch TV?" he asked.

"Nah. I'd rather just talk to you, if that's okay with you."

"Okay."

Minutes later he said he wanted to go to the bathroom.

"Why not just sit on your commode, Bert?" It was practically right next to his bed. "Then you won't have to walk all the way to the bathroom."

"No. Eleanor said she didn't want me using the commode, that it was too gross."

"I don't mind emptying it," I told him.

I took his arm and held it firmly as he walked slowly toward the bathroom, trailing his oxygen tube behind him. I had him stop several times so I could untangle the tube. By the time he reached the toilet, the tube was extended as far as it would go. I couldn't understand it. A considerable length of tubing was seemingly tangled up near the oxygen tanks, and upon close examination, I decided the tubing had been incorrectly connected. The tubing should have extended many more feet to allow Bert to go anywhere in the house he wanted.

Bert had me pull down his pajamas and assist him to sit on the toilet. Seconds after I went out and closed the door to give him privacy, he called me to help him up and to pull up his pajamas. Then I helped him walk back to his bed.

"Bert, I think you're walking better today than you did on Monday."

"Yeah. I feel better today."

"On Monday you were kind of unsteady on your feet. You even tried to get away from me once, remember?"

"Yeah," he laughed.

I also thought Bert seemed much less testy today than on Monday. He no longer was barking out orders like a drill sergeant.

Bert quickly invited me to look through several photo albums that included pictures taken during Eleanor's trip some years ago with some lady friends to Greece and Turkey, and pictures taken at their 50th wedding anniversary party; at his 75th birthday party; and at his 80th birthday and Eleanor's 73rd birthday party. The family gatherings were at their son Jake's house, which has a backyard swimming pool. The Greece and Turkey pictures were especially interesting to me because some were taken at well-known New Testament sites, including Patmos and Ephesus.

One of the albums also contained pictures of some Civil War mansions at Natchez, Mississippi, which Bert and Eleanor toured. Bert said he took the pictures with his camera that was "made in Germany."

After I looked at the albums, we chatted about various things, including the following:

- The family gatherings are at Jake's house, because of its size and its pool. It has five bedrooms, three baths, and two hot tubs, one indoors and one outdoors. Bert said the house cost $435,000, and that Jake, an extraordinarily handsome man in the pictures, is an executive at a large company. Jake is the oldest of their four children.
- Their daughter Amanda, next to oldest, lives in New York. She is a consultant. The pictures show her to have an extraordinarily beautiful face.

- Dan, next to youngest, repairs commercial appliances. He is handsome, like Jake.
- Rebecca, the youngest, works as a travel agent. She has a very pretty face, but of a different type of beauty than Amanda's.

"After looking at these pictures, I get the impression that Jake and Amanda are the aggressive ones, and that Dan and Rebecca are somewhat passive," I told Bert.

"You've hit it exactly. That's just the way they are."

"For heaven's sake! Is that right?"

Amanda is the only one of the four who has children (five), who have given Bert and Eleanor six grandchildren and 10 great-grandchildren.

- At one time Bert was vice president of manufacturing at a large company. He said he had 200 people working for him. The company made stainless steel sinks, urinals, stands, and other similar products. Now I understood why Bert tends to bark out orders like an Army sergeant: he was used to bossing a lot of people around.
- Bert said during the first two weeks he was put on hospice, his son Jake stayed with him while Eleanor went in for dialysis.

Bert and Eleanor are expecting their children this evening to celebrate her birthday.

At about 2:30 I called the oxygen company, asking them to come out and check Bert's tubing, which I thought hadn't been connected properly. While I was on the phone talking to them, Bert went to the bathroom and kept hollering for me. After I hung up, I went in the bathroom, and Bert was standing by the toilet. He couldn't get his pajamas down all the way. I pulled them down for him.

At 3:30, 15 minutes late, I remembered to give Bert the two pills Eleanor had set out for him.

At 3:45, about an hour after I called the oxygen company, their truck arrived. Harry and Doc, the truck's occupants, checked the oxygen tank and, at my urging, checked the tubing to Bert. They found it had indeed not been connected properly, and they reconnected it, giving Bert much more leeway to get around the house, especially to the bathroom. They left a new mask for Bert and showed me how to work the oxygen tank controls.

I asked them about the "oxygen" that drifted down the side of one of the tanks Monday after they had recharged it. They said it was merely water vapor and not oxygen, and that it was harmless and stops after a few minutes.

After they left I attached the new mask to the oxygen tube and put it around Bert's head. The mask seemed to fit much better than the old one, but it, too, kept slipping out of place. Connecting the hose to the mask required considerable finger dexterity.

At 4 o'clock Bert decided to lie down and rest, and he blew his nose on a tissue. He told me blood had come out. I looked at the tissue; indeed, it was tainted red. I wondered what that meant. Was it something I should be concerned with? I looked again at the tissue. I concluded it wasn't enough blood to worry about but made a mental note to monitor his discarded tissues.

Bert slept soundly from 4 until 4:20, snoring loudly. While he slept, I ate my "lunch": hot tea from my Thermos, three slices of rye bread, a handful of almonds and raisins, and a pear. When he awoke he asked me to get him some "fish" snacks from a box in the kitchen. I put some of the snacks into a small dish and brought this to him. Not being able to use his fingers because of his stroke, Bert spilled the snack onto the floor. I picked them up and put them back into the dish. Bert, however, said he no longer wanted them, and I left the dish on his tray.

I asked Bert what Eleanor was going to fix him for supper, and he said "popcorn shrimp."

At 4:20 Bert's niece called and chatted with him. She had just got back from Wisconsin.

Bert had me go to the kitchen and bring him a Baby Ruth candy bar three separate times. The candy bars were small, something like the kind passed out to children on Halloween. Each time I had to remove the wrapper and put the candy in his mouth. After each candy bar I let him sip water from a straw.

Bert didn't use his commode once today. Several times when he went to the bathroom, he stood up and urinated. One time he had a BM and asked me to help him up from the toilet and pull his pajama bottoms up. I asked if he had wiped himself, and he said yes, he was pretty sure he had. I took his word for it but wondered how he could have wiped himself, what with the damage left by his stroke.

At 5:30 Bert had me turn on the TV, and I got on the network news. When it concluded, I switched to the local news, and then to a public education channel.

At 6:20 Bert asked me to call the dialysis unit at the hospital and inquire whether or not Eleanor had left. I found the number and called. She had just left.

Eleanor arrived at 6:45, and I wished her a happy birthday first thing before I would forget. She apologized for her delay. At the dialysis unit they had a problem getting a cap off a plug. I suggested she provide Bert with an exercise ball for him to use to strengthen his fingers.

Friday, Visit 3

At 1:55 I parked in the lot of the vacant commercial building across the street from Bert's home. One car was already parked there. As I crossed the street, seeing the oxygen truck in the driveway, I stopped and opened a conversation with Harry. He said Bert had requested a portable oxygen tank so he could go to a wedding.

"He would need three ten-pound tanks, which are on order, but in Bert's condition, no way would he be able to go to that wedding."

He asked me if I was a home caregiver or "something like that." I explained I was a hospice volunteer. His trainee, Doc, was in the truck, and I said hello. I touched a frosted oxygen line and commented that it was real cold.

I rang the doorbell and Eleanor let me in. She was guiding Bert to the bathroom, walking behind him with her hands on his hips, as though she were steering him. It looked something like they were doing one of those dances seen at a wedding reception. I went into the family room, where Bert's bed was located, and about five minutes later they returned. I joked with them, and Eleanor said Bert had had a bad night, walking all around because he couldn't sleep.

I asked Eleanor about her dialysis process. "There are seventeen chairs in the dialysis room, and all are always filled, from five a.m. to five p.m."

I complimented her for her Greece and Turkey pictures. I assured her not to worry while she was gone, that she could trust me totally. She said she does. She left two pills for me to give to Bert after four o'clock, and she said to give him the morphine "squirt medicine" if he was in a lot of pain. She said Bert and I could have a piece of her birthday cake from her Wednesday evening family get-together. As she was leaving at 2:10, she pointed out to me where important phone numbers were located in the kitchen near the phone.

"Oh, one more thing," she told me, "if a real estate agent calls, tell them they can show the house."

Bert had stretched out on his hospital bed and had turned on the TV with his remote control. He had on another Bonanza rerun. I sat down at the table about 10 feet away. Bert quickly fell asleep, and I turned down the TV volume and started to read one of John Updike's short stories from his book, "Trust Me."

I glanced over at Bert. The bed's surface was about 30 inches off the floor, a comfortable height to permit Bert ease in getting on and off the bed. A wicker wastebasket with a clear plastic bag was on the floor next to a walker at the head of his bed.

Bert awoke shortly, and I moved my chair close to his bed and we began to chat.

"How about getting me a piece of Eleanor's birthday cake," he said.

I went into the kitchen and found the cake, still in its box, in the refrigerator. I took it out of the box. It looked delicious. Thick, dark chocolate frosting. I found two small dishes, two forks, and a knife and cut two small pieces for Bert and myself. I handed Bert his dish with the cake, and he tried to feed himself but gave up and asked me to feed him. I would give Bert a bite of his cake, and then give myself a bite of my piece. Every time I put a fork of cake in his mouth, I was struck by the smallness of his mouth.

"Hey, this cake is really good, Bert. Boy, this is my kind of devil's food cake."

"Yeah, it is good. How about getting me another piece," Bert said, after I fed him his last bite.

"Bert, that's the best idea I've heard all day. I'm going to have another piece, too," I laughed.

With my help, Bert sipped water through a straw with his cake, and I washed mine down with a cup of tea from my Thermos. I took the dishes and forks into the kitchen and washed them. I looked for a place to drain the dishes and couldn't find one of those dish receptacles. Then I noticed the automatic dishwasher. No wonder.

At about 3:30 Bert headed for the bathroom, dragging his oxygen tube behind him. About half way there he took off his oxygen mask. In the bathroom I turned on the light for him. I pulled down his navy blue pajamas and he sat down on the toilet. I stepped out of the bathroom for a few minutes until he called me. I helped him stand and pulled his pajama bottoms back up. I followed him closely as he walked by himself, barefoot, back to his bed. I put his oxygen mask back on him.

One of the standing oxygen tanks appeared to be tilting slightly. Upon close examination, I saw that the tank was not seated properly in its carriage. I pushed down on it and it snapped into place with a loud click.

I read Bert a half dozen or so jokes from my seniors joke book, and he laughed heartily after each one. He fell asleep, and I put the book away. He awoke minutes later and apologized for sleeping so much. "I guess I'm extra tired today because I was so restless last night. I walked around during the night trying to sleep in four different beds. My niece is coming over to spend the night so Eleanor can get some sleep. I guess I kept Eleanor awake most of the night. My niece is a nurse."

I took hold of each of Bert's hands, as though I were shaking hands. I had to peel back the fingers of his right hand, which were curled in somewhat from his stroke. "Show me how tightly you can squeeze my hands, Bert." I was surprised. He squeezed quite hard.

We chatted about various things:

- I asked Bert if he could still swallow good, and he said yes. He told me he had had a big breakfast this morning: toast, cereal, and juice.

- He said his hair was starting to grow back in, darker. I looked closely and I couldn't see any dark hair. I fibbed and told him, "Yeah, I think I can see some dark hair coming back in."

- He told me again how they were trying to sell this house and move to a condo.

- I read the instructions for the face mask. It said the string is supposed to go *below* the ears. I had been putting the string *above* Bert's ears. I didn't try sticking anymore Band-Aids on his mask to hold the mask to his face. Bad idea.

- In talking about his wife's trip to Greece and Turkey, which he said she made with several lady friends, Bert said he had never been overseas.

Bert said he was a proficient draftsman and had a drawing board in the basement where he made engineering drawings.

At 4:30 Bert asked me to fix him a cup of tea. I went into the kitchen and poured a cup of water in a pan and put it on the electric stove and figured out how to turn it on. I brought the tea to Bert in a cup with a wide saucer. I kidded him that if he spilled it on himself, he could sue me. He laughed and said he would never do that. After it cooled a bit, I helped him drink it, holding the cup to his mouth. He had me get him a Milky Way candy bar from the kitchen to eat with the tea.

At 5 o'clock I remembered to give Bert the pills Eleanor had told me to give him at 4. Bert said he wanted to sit out on his front porch. I thought this to be strange. Didn't he mean sit on his back porch? No, he meant the *front* porch. I helped him out the front door to the porch and put a chair out for him, and he sat on it for about 30 minutes, then wanted to go back inside. It was much more difficult for Bert to go *down* the single step to the porch than it was to get back *up*. I assisted him very carefully in both instances to make sure he didn't fall. While on the front porch, he verified to me that, yes, the tree in his front yard was a bur oak. He said he put siding on his house so he would no longer have to paint.

Back inside the family room I asked Bert about the beautiful stained-glass window on the north side of the room. He said he had made it, cutting each piece of glass, putting the pieces in channels, and soldering the channels. "I also made the stained-glass eagle in the living room and was recently offered four hundred and fifty dollars for it," he said.

Starting at about 6 o'clock, Bert kept telling me he was worried about Eleanor getting back. I recalled he had me call the dialysis center on Wednesday to find out if Eleanor had left. I wanted to discourage him from asking me to do this again and told him, "I predict Eleanor will walk in the front door at six-forty." This brought a smile to Bert, and he let it go at that. Actually, Eleanor walked in the door at 6:46.

I apologized to Eleanor for not giving Bert his medicine until 5 o'clock, and she thanked me for telling her, indicating she would give him his next medicine an hour after the designated time. I told her Bert and I each had two pieces of her cake and that I had made Bert a cup of tea. She seemed surprised about the tea.

Monday

All morning I was looking forward to sitting with Bert while his wife went to dialysis. I was hoping Eleanor still had some of that delicious devil's food cake in the refrigerator.

I told Dorothy I was going to have Bert tell me everything he was thankful for.

At 12:55 p.m. Eleanor called. "I just wanted to tell you not to come this afternoon because I had to have Bert taken to the hospital. He became rather agitated and I couldn't control him, so I called nine-one-one."

I thought, wait a minute, something wasn't right. Bert was on hospice, and she had him taken to the hospital? It was my understanding that hospice patients were never taken to the hospital. (I found out at a meeting of hospice volunteers about a month later that there is a provision in the hospice agreement where a patient can be taken to the hospital if circumstances warrant. Apparently the circumstances were there for Eleanor.)

Eleanor asked me for my address, which I gave to her. "But you don't have to send me a thank-you card. I enjoyed my visits with Bert," I told her. I let her know how I bragged to Dorothy (my wife) about how good that devil's food cake was and how I was looking forward to having another piece.

"There's still a piece in the refrigerator," Eleanor laughed. My mouth watered at the thought of it.

I suggested Bert may have had another stroke, which could have precipitated the agitation symptoms. I told Eleanor I would plan on coming to her house on Wednesday to sit with Bert, assuming he would be home from the hospital by then.

Wednesday

Since I had not heard from Eleanor, I didn't know if I was supposed to go to her house to sit with Bert. Was he still in the hospital? I called her house at 10 o'clock and got her recorder and left a message. I did this again at 11:55, 1, and 1:30. I called at 8 p.m. and got her recorder again, but this time I didn't leave a message. Obviously, Bert was still in the hospital.

Thursday

At 10:50 I phoned and Eleanor answered. She said Bert was still in the hospital and was heavily sedated. She was very apologetic for not calling me. She said she had been at the hospital and stayed overnight there with her daughter. She was looking for a full-time caregiver and wondered if I would be interested. I told her I couldn't do that, that I wasn't qualified, but I was willing to help out while she went for her dialysis. She was making calls inquiring about full-time caregivers and said they charge up to $100 a day.

Eleanor said Bert was incoherent much of the time, but last night he was nearly his normal self. I wanted to ask if that piece of devil's food cake was still in the refrigerator, but thought that would be tacky.

Friday

At 11:05 I called Eleanor, wondering if maybe Bert was home and if she wanted me to come at 2 o'clock so she could go to dialysis. She said Bert would be coming home from the hospital today, that I wouldn't be needed, that her son would be coming over. I told her I would call her Monday morning to see if she would need me for Monday afternoon.

Saturday

My wife and I had been out, and when we returned at 3:50 p.m., I played back a message on the recorder. Eleanor had called, saying that her husband had died Friday afternoon about an hour after he was brought home from the hospital. Her voice was broken and it sounded as though she was crying. She said his breathing suddenly became very labored, that he started gasping for breath, and he died. She told me memorial services for Bert would be at 10:30 a.m. Monday in St. Mary Anglican Church. The term, "memorial services," told me that no body would be at the services, that Bert's body was to be cremated.

Monday

This was a holiday, and my wife and I had been looking forward to going to a parade. We were especially excited because presidential candidate Texas Governor George W. Bush and Dick Cheney, his running mate, were going to be in the parade. I regretfully called our daughter Tricia and told her we wouldn't be coming because I wanted to attend Bert's memorial service.

I left my house at 10 o'clock heading for the church. I had never been inside the church, but I knew it was across the street from the park. But what I didn't know was that another church was also across the street from the park. I mistakenly eased my car into a space in the parking lot of the wrong church. After I realized my mistake, I decided to leave my car there and walk to St. Mary.

I found myself catching up with an elderly woman who had made the same mistake. I walked with her to St. Mary Church, each of us confessing our stupidity for parking next to the wrong church.

Entering the church vestibule I saw Eleanor, dressed in black, accepting condolences. I got at the end of the line and, looking around, recognized three of Bert's and Eleanor's children, Amanda, Rebecca, and Jake, from their pictures. Where was Dan? Minutes later I was pressing her hand with both of mine expressing my sorrow for her loss. Suddenly Pastor Robert, whom I had met Wednesday at the house, came up to me and shook my hand, calling me by name, telling me he was so glad to see me again. I moved away from Eleanor so she could continue to receive condolence wishers and entered the sanctuary. An organ in a choir loft was playing softly. Where should I sit? I looked around and decided to sit in the back off to the side. I entered a pew on the left side several rows from the back and sat down.

I looked straight ahead at the stained-glass window behind the altar. Jesus, wearing a flowing red cape, dominated the scene. Jesus held a lamb in his right arm and a shepherd's staff in his left hand. A fan high above at the cathedral ceiling turned slowly. I wondered how it could move much air. I suddenly became conscious of how slippery the pew seat was. Had it been waxed? I looked around at the stone walls, at the light-brown wood pews, at the wood beams. Side windows had long narrow slits. Three lighted candles rested on each end of the altar. A lighted Easter candle was near the altar. Red carpeting covered the aisle.

Minutes later Pastor Robert, with glasses and slightly graying hair, wearing a white alb and a green stole, began the service. "We welcome you in the name of the Lord Jesus Christ who has defeated sin, death, and the devil by His own death and His glorious resurrection. It is our earnest desire that this worship service may be an affirmation of the faith which all Christians have in the living Lord Jesus Christ. Therefore, we urge you to share in expressing the faith in which Bert lived and died by joining in praying, meditating, reading and listening to God's words of comfort and of promise. May God bless our worship as together we celebrate the joyous victory God gives to all who believe in Jesus Christ as Savior and Lord."

Then the organ began playing the melody for "My Course Is Run, Praise God, My Course Is Run." Although four stanzas were printed in the hand-out program, I could hear only Pastor Robert's voice singing. I'm in a church choir and was going to sing at my full voice, but somehow it didn't seem appropriate, so I merely whispered the words.

Next, Bert's and Eleanor's son Jake walked up to the altar microphone to give a eulogy for his dad. Jake was dressed in a dark suit, appearing every bit as handsome as he was in the pictures in the family room. Speaking in a strong and steady voice, he said, "Dad loved to laugh ...had a great smile ...a twinkle in his eye ...loved to tell jokes ...enjoyed life ...set high standards for all in the family ...loved his family ...his last years were his best ...loved to talk on the phone to his family." Jake concluded by reading "Remember Me," which he said his dad had read at his sister's funeral. The last line was, "If you always think of me, I'll never be gone." Jake's eulogy lasted only about five minutes.

Then Pastor Robert read Psalm 23, "The Lord is my shepherd ..." and Isaiah 40:28-31, "Hast thou not known? hast thou not heard, that the everlasting God, the Lord, the Creator of the ends of the earth, fainteth not, neither is weary? There is no searching of his understanding. He giveth power to the faint; and to them that have no might he increaseth strength. Even the youths shall faint and be weary, and the young men shall utterly fall; but they that wait upon the Lord shall renew their strength; they shall mount up with wings as eagles; they shall run, and not be weary; and they shall walk, and not faint."

The organ began to play the melody for "On Eagle's Wings," and once again only Pastor

Robert's voice could be heard. That is one of my favorite hymns, but I sung it quietly so as not to be obtrusive. The New Testament reading was from II Timothy 4:6-8, and the Gospel reading was from John 14:1-6.

Next Pastor Robert led the congregation in reciting the Apostles' Creed. I was struck by its close resemblance to the one I learned in an early grade at St. Mary's Grammar School in Phoenix, Arizona. Were the Anglicans that close to Catholics?

Then came Pastor Robert's sermon. "In my Father's house are many rooms ...Bert was a devoted husband, loving father, a skilled craftsman ...he was a child of God and knew Jesus as his Lord and Savior ...Bert was independent ...he liked to be in control ...dying is like a child falling asleep, the father comes in and carries the child to comfort. Our heavenly Father comes down and scoops us up ..."

Then Pastor Robert read Bert's obituary. Next came the hymn, "Jerusalem the Golden," with only Pastor Robert's voice being heard above the organ melody. The Lord's Prayer, Benediction, and Postlude concluded the service.

I watched as Eleanor and her children walked down the main aisle toward the vestibule to accept condolences from the congregation. I estimated that the church could seat about 300, and that it was perhaps one-third full. The pews began to empty from the front. I would be the last to offer condolences to Eleanor. I wanted to speak with her again.

The line moved surprisingly fast and within 15 minutes or so I stood before Eleanor as the last member of the congregation. She was so very glad to see me again and introduced me to her four children. I asked her to tell me about Bert's death.

"They brought Bert home from the hospital about noon on Friday. Dan (her son) and Rebecca (her daughter) were there. Bert was comatose, and about an hour after he was home, he experienced difficulty in breathing and died. Death came at about one-twenty."

"You didn't go to dialysis on Friday?" I asked.

"No, I skipped it that day."

I told Amanda and Rebecca how pretty they were, and I told Dan how highly Bert had spoken of him. Eleanor invited me to attend the lunch that was to follow, but I declined, telling her my wife was waiting for me.

Thursday

The hospice office called to assign me a new patient. I expressed surprise that Bert had been taken to the hospital and said it was my understanding that once a person was put on hospice, the person would never go back to a hospital. The office explained that under certain circumstances the hospice will arrange to have a patient taken to the hospital. In Bert's case, Eleanor couldn't handle him, and that is why the hospice arranged for him to go back to the hospital. I related that Bert was the first patient I had who really kept me busy. "But I liked being busy. It made me feel needed."

Tuesday

I received a thank-you card from Eleanor. The printed message read:

"Perhaps you sent a lovely card,
Or sat quietly in a chair
Perhaps you sent a floral piece,
If so we saw it there.
Perhaps you spoke the kindest words,
As any friend could say.
Perhaps you were not there at all,
Just thought of us that day.
Whatever you did to console our hearts,
We thank you so much whatever the part."

She penned a brief note: "You did so much more, thank you!"

Rusty

Visit 1

Late in the afternoon the hospice office called to assign me a new patient. The office cut me off; it had another call and would get back to me. Minutes later it called back. My new assignment: Hans, 93; Parkinson's and Alzheimer's; takes him a while to respond when spoken to; wife, Maude, needs help in dealing with him; wants a visitor so wife can get free; their house is next to a business, which they own.

I called the number for Hans and Maude, but got no answer. Thinking it might be a different area code, I called the hospice office back; I had the correct area code. I was told that Maude walks with difficulty, and it takes her a long time to get to the phone. I called back and this time she answered after one ring.

She had a pleasant voice. I wondered how old she was. Could she be as old as her husband — 93? She didn't sound that old. After I explained that the hospice office wanted me to drop over and see how I as a volunteer could be of help, we scheduled my first visit for 7 o'clock that evening.

At 6:55 I parked in the driveway in front of a two-car garage with separate one-car doors. No other car was in the driveway. It was a fairly large 1 1/2-story brick house on a corner lot. I stepped up onto a sidewalk and concrete stoop adjoining the driveway and knocked on the door. I later grew accustomed to calling this the back door. A woman's friendly voice said I should come in. I opened the unlocked aluminum door, turned left, went up half a dozen steps and turned to my right, entering a spacious kitchen. A woman, identifying herself as Maude, was sitting with her back to me at a table having coffee and cookies. I introduced myself, took out my hospice badge and showed it to her, and sat down opposite her.

I was struck immediately by her charm. She had nice features and a warm, motherly smile. I estimated her age to be about 77.

She said her husband was in bed in a nearby bedroom. She invited me to have coffee and cookies with her, but I declined. She said they have four children and six grandchildren. Her son Justin runs the business. I had glanced at it when driving past and thought it looked weather-beaten and not very prosperous.

Maude and her husband have lived here for 50 years. She said she is 87, and seemed flattered that I thought she was only about 77.

Her husband's health has been declining. Two months ago he could get around with a walker; now, he is bedridden. Four or five days ago he got out of bed, and she found him on the floor. Today he told her, "I think I'm going to die in this bed."

Maude said she has been trying to write a book about her life, an autobiography. She said she has a copy she could give me. She has been making daily journal entries for many years, dating back to her childhood. I told her maybe I could help her assemble it all into a book.

Then her son Justin entered the kitchen. He was a nice looking man with a business bearing. He scrutinized my hospice badge, and we chatted briefly, I told them a bit about myself. Justin said when he retires, he would like to be a hospice volunteer, too.

Justin said my interior car lights were on. I looked outside and saw two small lights on under the rearview mirror that were apparently map-reading lights. I went out to turn them off, but was unable to. I came back and told Justin I couldn't turn them off, that I wasn't going to worry about them.

I told them how I've written some manuscripts but have nothing published yet. I briefly described: the story of an Alabama priest; the adventure story involving a Christian, Jew, and Muslim; the story about a priest who is tempted by a woman.

Maude said her husband has a sister, 87, who used to work at a publishing company editing manuscripts. I told her I'd like to meet her.

They asked me if I would like to meet the hospice patient, and I said, yes, by all means. Maude got up and walked with difficulty, bent over. She has a spur on her spine that aggravates a nerve. She headed for a walker, with wheels, and proceeded to walk, straightening her back considerably.

I glanced out a kitchen window at my car and was gratified that the lights had gone out automatically.

We went to a hallway and turned right into the first open doorway, a bedroom, where Hans lay near two windows in a hospital bed. I greeted him with, "Hi, Hans," but Maude corrected me right away.

"He goes by the name of Rusty." I walked up to his bed, smiling big, and grasped his right hand with both of mine. I didn't let go of his hand, but stood there and held it firmly as I spoke to him.

Rusty and I hit it off immediately. I had him laughing. He was responding to me readily. I commented that he had brown eyes. I complimented him for his good head of hair, and I pointed out to him that I don't have any hair. He looked up at me and said, "Yes, you do. I see one, two, three, four, five, six . . .," and we all burst out laughing.

"Rusty is sharp mentally," I told Maude and Justin. "The hospice office said he has Alzheimer's and Parkinson's. But I don't think he has Alzheimer's. I notice a tremor in one of his hands, and I suppose that means he has a touch of Parkinson's." I laughed. "I've got to stop playing doctor. Every time I play doctor I get myself in trouble." I laughed again.

Justin agreed that he didn't think his father had Alzheimer's.

I told them I would bring my old-folks joke book and read some jokes to Rusty. I asked him if he liked jokes, and he smiled and said yes. I told them how I've read this joke book to several other hospice patients.

I asked them who cuts Rusty's hair, which seemed a bit long. They said a friend comes over and does it.

I commented how nicely trimmed Rusty's fingernails are; Maude said she trims them.

I asked her how tall Rusty is and how much

he weighed in his prime. He looked so small. She said he is 5 foot 6 and always weighed about 135 pounds.

Justin, apparently satisfied he had checked me out sufficiently, excused himself and left.

I tried to show Rusty how to work the remote switch to raise and lower the head and foot ends of his bed. I pressed his finger on the six buttons: raise head, lower head, raise feet, lower feet, raise entire bed, lower entire bed. He didn't seem to grasp a thing I said.

I said good-bye to Justin, and Maude gave me a quick tour of the house, going counterclockwise: living room (large), with lots of family pictures; Maude's bedroom, large; a bathroom; a small bedroom (used by Maude as a sewing room); another small bedroom (used as a guest room); and the kitchen.

Maude and I went back into the kitchen, and we sat down at the table and chatted some more. She had an obvious preference for the chair on the east side of the table, with her back to the sink. I once again sat in the chair on the other side of the table, facing her. She got me a copy of her life's story for me to take with me. She brought me her current journal book and asked me to read a page or two. I told her I'd read it next time.

We set 3 o'clock Friday for my next visit. She seemed pleased.

When I left, it was 8:10. When I got home I read Maude's life story: 2 1/2 pages, single-spaced. I then re-read it, making copious notes so I could understand it. Here is a copy of that story (with names changed):

I have just passed a milestone at the age of 80 years. Life passes by so rapidly it's difficult to understand what happened as the end approaches.

My earliest recollections are of farm life in a suburb of a large city, perhaps between the ages of 3-5. This happy existence came to an end in 1918 at age 5 when my mother, stepfather and half brother died during the flu epidemic. I don't understand why I was spared, but that left my brother William, who was visiting our Aunt Beth, my mother's sister in Wisconsin at the time, and me to face the world. We weren't alone, however, as Aunt Beth took us to her home. There with her and Uncle Jack, we had a good home and a secure future, until one night one year later Aunt Beth was taken from us with a heart attack.

My mother's brother, Don, was assigned as our guardian and he decided we should live with our paternal grandmother in a large city. Once again we had a home, but not a very stable one. I loved Grandma but it seems she had too great an interest in our inheritance from the sale of the farm and was constantly after Uncle Don for more money—even taking him to court and causing his loss of wages. This led him to decide we would be better off in an orphanage and we would have a religious education. In retrospect, I think *it was right, for Grandma ended her life in a county hospital without a cent. We had each other but the boys and girls in the orphanage were restricted from socializing, so we didn't see one another very often. We spent five long years there and dreamed of a home—any home!*

William graduated from grade school and was farmed out to a florist in another suburb. At this time, Uncle Don took me to live in his home nearby. I lived with his family for 2 years while I finished grade school. It was not a very happy home since they had 3 daughters ages 8, 12 and 18. The eldest daughter was very kind, but the other two not so. Then Aunt Maggie, in her 40's became pregnant and they decided I was too much to take care of. So back to the orphanage I went. Then I was placed with some elderly farm folks with 3 grown-up children (2 married daughters and a 28 year old son). There was plenty of work on the farm. I spent the time there in 1927 from June to Oct. when all the harvesting was finished and I was no longer needed. I went back to the orphanage to wait for another, what was called "mother's helper" job. I was placed with a family with 2 small children ages 2 and 4 and another on the way. My job in the beginning was to get up in the morning, change the baby, and dress the other two. Later as time went on, I was taught to make Mr. Trent's breakfast and clean up the table and dishes. As time went on, Mrs. Trent very cleverly taught me the rudiments of housekeeping at which I became very efficient. Soon, my job was to do everything—cooking, cleaning, ironing, and taking care of the children. The responsibility of all this was quite a load and I felt I was being taken advantage of, especially since I was paid nothing except a dollar to take in a movie now and then.

The great depression was on at that time and Mrs. Trent complained she couldn't afford me any more. My brother was working at his third job then and living with a family with 10 children. They hired him to help with business and field work. He fell in love with one of the girls and planned marriage around the time I was thinking of leaving the Trents, so William found a place for me with his fiancé's Aunt Kate in 1932. There I had the opportunity of completing 1 year of high school at age 19. In the meantime, William married and took me as a permanent boarder (not too permanent). He rented a truck farm and I came in handy in the field hoeing, weeding, cultivating, and harvesting the crops for market in 1933. It seemed that's where I belonged (on a farm).

After three years there, I married my sister-in-law's brother and moved to a nearby suburb. We had a little 2 room house to go to which was our own—

bought and paid for with my inheritance. Rusty's father donated a new hardwood floor and William did most of the painting. We had no running water, just electricity and outdoor plumbing, but indoor plumbing came later when Rusty built 2 bedrooms and a bathroom in the attic. Then a large kitchen was added and a garage. We were blessed with 4 children so it was beginning to get crowded and Rusty began building our present home in 1948. This was in the building until 1950 when we sold our honeymoon home and moved to our present home. The children were Justin - 14; Janet - 11; Richard - 9, and Charlotte - 2. Justin and Janet didn't stay very long in our new home for both married at age 20. Charlotte went off to college after high school and met Harvey. They married and had 2 children and moved to another state.

Here, I had more time and could help a little more with Rusty's business. Rusty and William formed a partnership and that lasted until 1953 when William died after suffering a fall. His wife remained in the partnership for about 5 years. She then remarried and we bought the business from her. The market for the business was dwindling, so we gradually went into growing garden flowers and vegetables. We did very well and built a business which we turned over to Justin in 1980 since we were then 73 and 67. They (Justin and

Cassie, his wife) built the business to where it is now—very successful.

It is now 1994. We're nearing the end of our sojourn on this earth and hope for the best for our children. Rusty is 87 and I am 81. (Story modified slightly to remove dates and names of cities)

Signed,

Maude

One Day Later, Visit 2

Maude was walking from her open garage toward the back door at 2:55 when I parked in the driveway. She was stooped over and obviously just barely able to walk. I got out of the car quickly and went up to her just as she was opening the back door. I spoke to her, but she said she wasn't able to turn around and look at me. She reminded me to close the door because the air-conditioning was turned on. I followed her up the steps and into the kitchen.

We exchanged a few pleasantries, and I returned her mini-autobiography to her, taking it out of the envelope. She told me to leave it in the envelope, as that is where she keeps it. I told her I would like to read one of her journals.

"You're here to see Rusty, so let's go and see him," she said.

"All right. But I'm also here to see you and to help you. Have you figured out how to use me?"

"Well, I don't know."

"Does Justin (her son who runs the business) look in on you periodically?"

"Yes. He was here this morning, and again at noon. And he stops by in the evening."

"That's good. Did the nurse and nurse's aide come today?"

"Yes. The nurse's aide comes Monday through Friday and gives Rusty a bath. The nurse came this morning too and checked him over. She said he's doing real good."

I went into Rusty's room by myself, as Maude said she was going to get a couple of her journals for me to look at.

"Hi, Rusty," I said as cheerfully as I could. He was lying on his back, with the head of the bed elevated considerably. He had on a navy blue T-shirt with the "C" emblem for a baseball team. The only other thing he had on was his diaper. His brown blanket was down around his knees, and he was making an effort to reach the blanket.

"Would you like me to take the blanket off?"

"Yes."

I picked up the blanket and tossed it on the nearby bed.

"Who are you?" Rusty asked.

"You don't remember me?"

"No. Should I remember you?"

"I was here last night, Rusty. My name is Joe. You don't remember?"

"No. You were here last night?"

"Yes. I see you're wearing a shirt with the emblem for a baseball team."

"Huh?" He had no idea what I was talking

about.

"Do you like jokes, Rusty?"

"Yes," he smiled.

"Okay. I brought along my joke book. I'll read you a joke." I picked up my joke book, which pokes good-natured fun at senior citizens. I began looking for a simple joke that perhaps Rusty could understand.

Maude entered the room, leaning on her walker, which had four wheels. She had two journal books in the basket of the walker. She sat down in a nearby chair and began to look through one of the books.

"I don't think Rusty will understand if you read him a joke," she said.

"I think you're right." I closed the book and set it down.

"Oh, this is so boring," Maude said, referring to her journaling.

I picked up a journal book and started to read. I couldn't believe it. She was right. There were statements like, "I did a lot of laundry today. It was a nice day. The high temperature was 85. The sun rose at 5:37 and set at 8:21." I had looked forward to reading her journals and, if they were good, to help her compile them into a manuscript, with the purpose of perhaps getting it published.

"I have a real old journal. The first one I ever kept. I'll get it," she said. She headed out of the room, leaning on her walker.

I was determined to get a conversation going with Rusty.

"What is your favorite flower, Rusty?" I thought this would be a good question, since he had worked in a business for much of his life.

"My favorite flower? I don't know," he laughed.

Well, I struck out on that.

"What is your favorite tree?"

"I don't know," he laughed again.

"Who was William?" I asked. I knew that William was Maude's brother; that Rusty and William had been partners in the business; and that William had died in a fall.

"Who was William? He was Maude's brother." I thought that was pretty good. He has a memory after all!

Maude came back into the room, stooped over without her walker, and sat down.

"Here's my old journal book. Somebody gave it to me as a gift back about 1930. Oh, but I don't have the key. I need to get the key for it." She looked around for her walker.

"Where is my walker?"

"I'll go find it for you." I found it in her bedroom and returned it to her.

She leaned onto the walker and said she was going to look for the key to unlock the diary.

I tried striking up another conversation with Rusty. Maude returned quickly.

"I found the key," she said, leaving the walker and sitting down. She unlocked the diary and started paging through it.

"I haven't looked at this in years. Gee, my entries weren't very good."

"When did William die?" I asked.

"When he was forty-two. He fell from a roof and struck his head on a pipe."

"Oh, how terrible! Such a young age. Did he have children?"

"Yes. A boy and a girl. One was in college and one was in high school."

"How much older that you was William?"

"Three years."

I looked at Rusty and it struck me suddenly that he didn't look very comfortable.

"I think I'll try to make him more comfortable," I told Maude.

"Put his blanket back on him."

"Rusty, do you want your blanket back on you?"

"Yes."

"Okay." I spread it over his legs and diaper. I lowered the head of his bed and reached under both of his arms and tugged him forward about a foot or so. I raised his head and fluffed his pillow. Then I straightened out the sheet he was lying on.

"There, Rusty, now you look comfortable."

I raised the head of his bed a little ways and stopped.

"How's that, Rusty? Is that better?"

"Yes," he smiled.

"Tell me about yourself," Maude said suddenly.

"I was sort of an orphan just like you were." I told her how my parents had split up when I was 3 1/2 and how I had been deposited at a Catholic sisters' convent in Phoenix, Arizona.

"How long did you stay there?"

"Until I was ten."

"Then what happened to you?"

"I was put in four different foster homes and finally to Boys Town. Have you heard of Boys Town?"

"Sure. That was a good movie. Was it like the movie?"

"Well, sort of."

"Spencer Tracy won an Academy Award for his role as Father Flanagan," she said.

Her memory impressed me.

"Well, have you figured out how to use me?"

"Can you fix things?"

"Sure."

"Could you tighten up the toilet seat? It's real loose."

"Sure." I went to the bathroom and checked the toilet seat. It was indeed very loose. I finger-tightened the nuts for the seat, but I needed a screwdriver to complete the job. Maude said she had one in a kitchen drawer. Minutes later I finished the job, making the seat about as secure as was humanly possible. While fixing it, I couldn't help but notice some loose ceramic tile behind the toilet.

"There. It's all fixed," I smiled.

"Oh, thank-you so much."

"Anything else I can fix?"

"I'd like to have new door handles put on both doors. Do you know how to do that?"

"Sure. I'd be happy to. Listen, I think I have a

feel now how I can be of help to you. How about if I come back on Monday and bring some tools, and fix some things for you."

She laughed. "You must have enough things to fix at your own house."

"Oh, yeah, I do. But that's okay. I can fix some things for you, too."

I thought suddenly to ask her what color eyes she had.

"My eyes are a blue-gray."

"And, Rusty's eyes are brown, aren't they?"

"Oh, yes. His have always been the deepest brown."

I asked her what part of Europe Rusty's grandparents came from, and she said Rusty didn't know. I told her my father's family came from Baden-Baden, Germany.

"That's where so many Jews were taken away to be killed. I read a story about it."

"Is that right?" Then I remembered. When I was a Navy electronics instructor, one of my students was named Schrantz, and he said he was Jewish. Maybe my Schrantz German ancestors also were Jewish. Yet, I was raised Catholic and was told that my German ancestors were Catholic.

I checked my watch, and it was four o'clock. I had been there a little over an hour. I wanted to leave so I wouldn't be going home in heavy traffic.

"I think I had better be going." I grasped Rusty's hand with both of mine. "Good-bye, Rusty. I'll see you on Monday."

"Good-bye," he smiled. I wondered if he still

remembered who I was.

Maude got up and leaned on her walker and accompanied me through the kitchen. I went down the steps and looked at the back door. "Is this the handle you want me to replace?"

"Yes. I want to get a handle with a lock on it."

I looked at the latch, and it did indeed lack a lock.

"Oh, never mind, I can get Justin to replace them."

"Okay. Well, good-bye, Maude. I'll see you at two o'clock on Monday."

"Okay. Good-bye."

Three Days Later, Visit 3

I arrived at 1:50, and the weather appeared to be very threatening, with dark clouds gathering in the northwest. It was warm (89) and very humid. Possible severe thunderstorms were forecast for later in the afternoon. I parked in the driveway, and the garage door was open. I got out of the car toting my toolbox, opened the screen door, knocked on the inner door, but heard no response. I opened the inner door and called Maude a couple of times, but got no answer. I went inside, up the stairs to the kitchen, calling for Maude. I set my toolbox on the kitchen table. Not seeing her, I went into the hallway and turned to the right into Rusty's room. Maude was lying on the bed on her left side facing Rusty. Rusty was on his right side in his bed facing Maude. Both appeared to be asleep. I went into the room and softly spoke Maude's name, and she answered me and got up, and Rusty said hello.

"Did I wake you?" I asked Maude.

"No, I wasn't asleep," she said, sitting up on the side of the bed.

"Hello, Rusty," I smiled, grasping his hand.

"Hello," he said, not having any idea who I was.

"He doesn't remember you," Maude said.

"That's okay. Hi, Rusty. My name is Joe."

"Hi, Joe," he smiled.

Maude stood up and leaned on her stroller and headed for the kitchen.

"I've lost one of my hearing aids," she said. "I wear one in each ear, and the one I lost works best and is my favorite."

"I'll help you look for it," I volunteered.

"I've looked in all the usual places and I can't find it. The darn thing cost $1,300, too."

"Wow! Then I better look real hard for it and find it for you," I said.

I told her how I recently found the lower false teeth lost by an Alzheimer's patient.

"I love to look for things," I added. "Could you take out your remaining hearing aid so I can see just what it is I'm looking for?"

She removed the hearing aid from her left ear and set it on the table.

"Boy, that is really small, isn't it? That lost hearing aid is going to be hard to find!" I said.

"The lost one goes in my right ear, and that's the ear that really needs a hearing aid."

We set out on a search for the hearing aid.

With her permission, I looked everywhere I could think of: in the kitchen, in Rusty's bedroom, in the living room, in Maude's bedroom, in the bathroom, in the sewing room, and in the guest bedroom. I couldn't find it anywhere. I got down on my hands and knees, searching the floor.

"Maude, I give up. I've looked everywhere."

"All right. I'll just keep looking. If I don't find it I'll just have to buy another one."

I asked Maude if I could get the mail for her.

"Sure. But if the red flag is still up, that means it hasn't come yet."

I went outside and checked the mailbox. It was alongside the road at the intersection. The red flag was still up, and the sky looked more threatening than ever. A storm was imminent. I went back inside.

Maude went into the sewing room and began to sift through a pile of paperback books.

"Are you going to throw these out?" I asked.

"Most of them. Would you go down in the basement and bring up a box to put them in?" she asked.

"Sure."

I went downstairs and found a big cardboard box and brought it up to the room. She was bending over, going through the books, forming two piles: the ones she wanted to keep and the ones she didn't want. She had me put the ones she didn't want into the box.

"You can have any of those you want," she said, indicating the ones in the pile she didn't want.

"Okay." I set aside seven Agatha Christie books for my wife, and about half a dozen books for myself. I put the discards in the box and carried the ones I wanted out to my car. The storm was practically upon us.

"You can have that old bookcase if you want it," Maude said, pointing to an inexpensive-looking metal bookcase.

"Okay. But it's too big for me to get into my car. But maybe if I could take it apart." I quickly knocked it apart and stacked the shelves and sides in a pile and carried them out to the car. I could hear thunder off to the northwest where the sky was black.

"Does your wife have small feet?" she asked suddenly.

"Yeah, as a matter of fact, she does," I said.

"Well, why don't you take these slippers home for her. I bought them for myself, but they're too small."

"Okay." I put them in my toolbox so I wouldn't forget them. They were kind of cute, with zebra-like stripes.

Maude sat down in her easy chair in the living room to turn on the TV and watch for a weather forecast. I remained standing.

"You sure are a nervous creature," she said.

I felt myself trying to stop all physical activity just to show her I really wasn't so nervous after all. I marveled that she had called me a "creature." I moved a chair close to her and sat down to chat, trying to sit as still as possible to hide my apparent nervousness. About 15 minutes later it appeared the storm was practically upon us, and I went outside to check the mail again. The red flag was down. I went to the mailbox and brought in two letters, both junk mail: something from the Silesian Fathers and from Bose Radio. She opened the Silesian envelope right away and said she likes to get mail from them because they send her little prayer leaflets. Sure enough, one was enclosed. She said she had sent them some money a few years ago, and they're always writing her and asking for more. But she wasn't going to send them any more.

We talked about Rusty.

"He wants to go, but is afraid to," she said.

"You mean, he wants to die but is afraid to?"

"Yes."

"When he was put on hospice, did they give an estimate about how much longer he would live?"

"No. But the fact that they put him on hospice means they don't expect him to live more than six months," she said.

"Does he eat well?"

"No. He used to, but lately he hasn't been eating much at all."

I wanted to tell her that before hospice people die, they stop eating. But I didn't think it appropriate to tell her that.

"Does he drink liquids good?"

"No. He just drinks a little bit."

Suddenly it began to lightning and thunder, and a driving rain lashed the house. How we needed the rain!

"I would like to repair the ceramic tile in the bathroom, Maude," I said. "Would that be all right?"

"You know how to do that?"

"Sure."

"Okay. Some of the tiles are broken. You can go downstairs and see if you can find some tile. I know there are some down there."

I went downstairs and couldn't believe how fast I found them. On a table against a wall was a small box containing odds and ends, including half a dozen ceramic tiles exactly matching the ones in the bathroom. I brought them upstairs and showed them to Maude.

"They are a perfect match," I said exuberantly. I set them down on the bathroom sink counter. "When I come back next time, I'll repair the tile for you. I'll have to pick up some ceramic adhesive and some grout."

We sat back down in the living room. The rain was pounding against the windows. Maude told me about her children, and she talked about her husband. Things I learned included:

- Her son Richard was driving to Maryland, and Maude was expecting a call from him. She said he had told her he would call her as soon as he got there.
- Maude had recently given Richard her car, a 1993 Ford with only 8,000 miles on it.
- Richard is autistic. He lived with his mother until recently, when he left home to move in with a friend.

Maude said Rusty swears when she tries to talk religion to him. She doesn't know if he believes in an after life.

Later we went into the kitchen to talk. She sat facing a TV and turned it on to get the weather. A weather alert began to flash across the screen, warning that severe thunderstorms were expected until 3:30. It was then 3:20.

Maude poured a glass of orange juice for Rusty. I carried it into his room for her, and she followed, leaning onto her walker. I raised the head of Rusty's bed so he could drink it. As she brought the glass to his mouth, he brought his hands up and grasped the glass. Maude gradually let go, and he started to drink it by himself.

"Gee, he drinks good, doesn't he!" I said.

He slowly but steadily drained the glass, not spilling a drop.

When Maude and I returned to the kitchen, I told her our small grandchildren drink out of what I called toddler glasses with a protrusion on the lid to suck from. She asked me if I would bring her one of those for Rusty.

When I had been in the bathroom checking the tile, I noticed that the ceiling exhaust blower grill was very dusty. I told her I was going in the bathroom to clean it. I took along a step-stool from the kitchen. As I was in the process of cleaning it, her son Justin entered the bathroom. We exchanged greetings, and I told him what I was doing, that I was going to repair her tile for her. He went to the bathtub to examine the tile.

"I see that some of those have beveled edges," he said.

"They do?" I looked. Sure enough. "Justin, I'm so glad you pointed that out. I hadn't noticed. You're right, one side of those damaged tiles has a beveled edge. I'll have to go to the tile store and see if I can pick up some with a beveled edge."

When I finished with the exhaust blower, I picked up my toolbox and told Maude I was leaving. "I can't come back until Thursday," I told her.

"Anytime."

"Okay. I'll see you about one o'clock Thursday afternoon."

Three Days Later, Visit 4

I arrived at about 1:30, parked in the driveway, and entered through the back door without ringing the bell.

"Hello!" I called out, walking up the stairs to the kitchen. I didn't hear a reply and when I didn't see anyone in the kitchen, I repeated the "Hello" several times, and went into Rusty's bedroom, where Maude was standing by his bed.

"I brought you a couple of things, Maude."

"You did? What did you bring me?" she smiled.

I handed her a clear plastic bag of four tomatoes.

"You can take those back home with you. I can't eat tomatoes. They're bad for my arthritis," she said matter-of-factly.

"Okay. And here are a couple of those plastic child glasses I was telling you about. The ones with the lids with a protuberance for the child to suck from. Maybe you can find it useful to give Rusty his drinks out of these."

"Thank-you. I'll try them. They ought to

eliminate the spillage. When I give him a drink from a glass, I usually spill some on him."

"Oh, and one more thing," I said. "I went to the tile store with a sample of your tile to see if I could replace the fourteen pieces of tile at the back of your bathtub. They said your tile pattern has been discontinued. So I didn't buy any. You'll have to tell me what to do."

"You can tell Justin and let him decide."

Coincidentally, Justin entered the bedroom.

"Are you ready to go?" he asked Maude.

Maude said she was ready, that Justin was going to take her to a supermarket. She asked me if I would mind staying with Rusty and feed him lunch while she went to the store with Justin.

"I would love to," I told her.

I quickly told Justin that the tile store said Maude's bathroom tile pattern had been discontinued and asked him what I should do.

"Get fourteen tiles that you think match as closely as possible," he said.

Maude warmed up Rusty's lunch in the microwave oven. "You can give him this," she told me. I looked at the plate. It contained ground liver, mashed potatoes, green beans, and one slice of buttered white bread. She poured some milk into one of the plastic glasses that I brought, and I put on the lid.

Rusty had slipped down somewhat in his bed, and Maude asked me to pull him forward so I could feed him. Although Rusty is small, I thought he was pretty heavy when I tugged at him.

"I see Rusty now has a catheter," I told Maude.

"Yes. Now I won't have to change his diaper as often."

The urine in the clear plastic bag was very dark. I wondered if that was because he was dying or simply because he was in his 90's.

Maude and Justin left, and I began feeding Rusty. He ate quite well, finishing almost everything, including the slice of bread and his milk. But he didn't suck from the child's lid very good, and I removed the lid and let him drink from the rim of the glass. He drank nicely without any spillage.

When I finished feeding him, I thought the air in his bedroom smelled foul, as if he might have had a BM. I opened the window by the foot of his bed, and the fresh air felt good.

With Rusty fed, I went into the bathroom and set about removing the four pieces of "loose" tile from the wall near the floor behind the toilet. Rusty kept interrupting me with grunting sounds, and each time I went to his bedside to see if anything was wrong. Once I adjusted his blanket, which seemed to please him.

Pretty soon Maude and Justin returned, with Justin bringing in her groceries and placing them on the kitchen table. I had Justin come into the bathroom so I could show him the slight progress I had made in removing those four tiles behind the toilet. He seemed eager to get back to the business and left shortly.

I told Maude I thought Rusty had loaded his diaper. She opened the window and looked inside his diaper. "There's nothing in it. It was just gas." She had me get a fan from her room and bring it in to Rusty's room, set it on the floor, plug it in and turn it on to get rid of the foul smell.

Then I set about in earnest to remove the four tiles. It was really hard to do. The tile appeared to be loose, and at first I thought their removal would be easy. But each tile had a thick layer of some dried-up sticky, gooky material with part of the material still sticking to the wall. I finally got them off, but only after taking off some of the wall plaster. I took them out to the driveway to scrape off the material, whatever it was.

Scraping off that material was a real job! Why was I doing this? What had I got myself into? As a hospice volunteer, wasn't I just supposed to sit with the patient? To prevent breaking the four squares of tile, I had to position them flat on the driveway while scraping off that sticky material. With a sharp chisel-like tool in my right hand, and my left hand holding the tile, I went about my task. It wasn't long before I accidentally jabbed my left thumb under the nail with the tool causing the thumb to begin bleeding. Oh, brother! I took out my handkerchief and wrapped the thumb and continued working. But it really did hurt!

Finally, I got most of that awful sticky material off the tile. I took them into the bathroom and placed them on the right end of the long sink counter. Then I got out my can of wood filler and putty knife and filled in the holes in the plaster where I had removed the tile. The lower portion of the four pieces of tile had been installed about half an inch below the floor line. I thought that was strange, and filled in that depression with the wood filler. When I was through, the substrate looked nice and smooth, ready to receive the tile once again. But in filling in that floor depression, I inadvertently created a new problem, which I was to find out about tomorrow.

I asked Maude not to disturb the newly leveled area where I had removed the tile. "I need to let it dry for twenty-four hours," I told her. "I'll come back tomorrow and reattach those four pieces of tile." But I had a surprise coming.

I couldn't do anything more in the bathroom so I went into Rusty's bedroom and sat by his bed and started talking to him.

"Do you remember my name, Rusty?"

"No," he said decisively.

"Do you know the names of your children?" I asked.

"No," he said just as firmly.

"Your children's names are Justin, Richard, Janet, and Charlotte."

He was unimpressed, showing no sign of recognizing the names.

I began to study Rusty's profile. I was struck by how Jewish he looked. I thought he had a beautiful nose profile. But, oh, how Jewish. The tip of his nose dipped slightly.

I began to study his head structure. He had wide jawbones, like me. Could my ancestors and Rusty's ancestors have emigrated from the same part of Germany? I was willing to bet they had. Maybe Rusty and I were distant cousins once or twice removed.

I began to get discouraged trying to chat with him. He just plain had no idea what I was talking about. So I went into the kitchen, where Maude was sitting at the table working a crossword puzzle.

"I'm going to interview a caregiver for Rusty tomorrow," she said.

"You are?" Wait a minute. If she was going to bring in a caregiver, that wouldn't leave anything for me to do for Rusty. Oh, well. I could still fix things around the house for Maude.

"They charge ten dollars an hour," she said.

"They do? Twenty-four hours a day?"

"I think so."

"Wow! That will get expensive real fast. Say, did you ever find your hearing aid?"

"No," she laughed.

It was 4:10 and I got up to leave.

"Would you mind getting me a wastebasket for Rusty's room?"

"A wastebasket for Rusty's room? Sure, I can do that. What kind do you want?"

"It doesn't make much difference. Preferably one I can put his diapers in, with a lid so his bedroom won't smell."

"I'll be only too happy to," I told her.

The Next Day, Visit 5

I parked in the driveway at 1:30. Carrying the new wastebasket I had bought for Maude, I knocked on the back door, went inside, calling out, "Maude." Seeing no one in the kitchen, still calling out "Maude," I went into the hallway. Entering Rusty's bedroom, I saw that Maude was lying on her left side on the double bed facing Rusty's hospital bed. Rusty saw me and said, "Someone's here."

Maude opened her eyes and began to make an effort to sit up. "Hi, Maude. Don't get up. Stay there and finish your nap. I'll go ahead and get to work in the bathroom. I brought you a wastebasket. I hope you like it."

I held it up to show her, and she sat up to see it.

"It's just like the kind we have at home. It has a lid on it that opens and closes."

"Yes, that will be fine. I need a lid to keep the diaper smells from getting out."

"I think you had told me to get one with some color, but all the store had was white."

"White will be fine," she smiled, inspecting the wastebasket.

I turned to Rusty. The head of his bed was partially raised, and he was lying on his back with his knees sticking up.

"Hi, Rusty."

"Hi," he said without smiling, as though he knew me.

"Who am I, Rusty?"

"I don't know," he said matter-of-factly.

"I'm Joe-Joe from Kokomo," I smiled.

"Joe-Joe from Kokomo," he repeated.

"You don't remember me, huh?"

"No. Should I?"

"No, you don't have to remember me. That's okay. I'm Joe-Joe from Kokomo."

"Joe-Joe from Kokomo," he echoed.

Maude left the room for the kitchen.

"Well, Rusty, I have to get into the bathroom and get to work on those tiles."

I went out to my car and returned with my little red plastic toolbox, a recent birthday gift from our daughter Tricia.

Returning to the house and the kitchen, I told Maude, "I'm going to put those tiles back on, the ones I took off behind the toilet at the floor." She appeared to be preparing herself something to eat.

In the bathroom I picked up the four tiles from which I had so laboriously scraped off that awful sticky stuff, damaging my left thumb. I bent down by the toilet with the intention of going through the motions of making sure they would fit before I applied the tile adhesive.

What the dickens! Not one of the tiles would fit! I had filled in the ridge below the floor line with wood filler, effectively making the tiles too long. No way did they fit! Oh, brother! Now what do I do? I would have to scrape out most of the wood filler from that ridge. I tried scraping it. It wasn't going to budge. It was as hard as a rock! Oh, boy! I'll have to take these tiles somewhere and have them cut.

I measured the tiles and the allotted space for them between the other tiles on the wall and the floor. The tiles were now a half inch too long. I would need half an inch cut from each of them!

I dejectedly went into the kitchen and

explained my problem to Maude.

"You can take them to Ace Hardware and they can cut them for you."

"Okay." I took the four pieces of tile out to my car so I wouldn't forget them.

I went back into the bathroom and removed the 14 tiles from the horizontal ledge at the back of the bathtub and prepared the substrate, applying some wood filler to smooth it out. Half of these tiles were broken, which I put into the wastebasket. Then I removed six loose tiles from the wall in front of the tub and prepped that substrate.

Next I took the 13 squares of tile out to the driveway and proceeded to scrape away the old adhesive. This was a much easier task than dealing with that awful sticky stuff from the four tiles behind the toilet. I soon had them clean, being careful not to break the tiles and not to gouge my thumb again. I returned the tiles to the bathroom, placing them on the right side of the sink counter.

I went into the kitchen and told Maude I couldn't do anymore with the tiles until tomorrow.

"I forgot to tell you the bathtub soap dish is loose. Do you think you could fix it?" she smiled.

"I can sure try. Sometimes that can be a real challenge. I'll go take a look at it."

I was able to pull the ceramic fixture out of the wall. I cleaned it up a bit, applied a thick coat of adhesive around it, and pushed it back into the hole in the wall, holding it in place for a few minutes to let it set. When I let go, it remained firmly in place. There! That little job is done, and without complications! I went into the kitchen and told Maude, who was still sitting at the kitchen table.

"You're just a real fix-it man, aren't you? How much am I going to owe you?"

"How much are you going to owe me? Nothing for my labor. Just for any materials I have to buy," I smiled. I handed her a receipt for the wastebasket. "It cost me thirteen dollars and forty-nine cents."

She went to her bedroom and returned with her purse and peeled out a 10-dollar bill and four singles. I returned her two quarters and a penny, but she insisted I keep them "for a tip."

She looked at me strangely. "I've never met anyone like you before," she said.

I went into Rusty's bedroom to chat with him again. The conversation was a repeat of the one I had with him before. He again didn't know who I was. Maude came into the room and asked me to pull him forward again. This time I lowered the head of his bed and got behind his head and reached forward under his arms and tugged him toward me. That technique simplified the task considerably.

"I hired a full-time caregiver, a woman. She starts tomorrow," Maude said. "She charges ten dollars an hour, even when she sleeps," she laughed.

"Even when she sleeps? Boy! That's going to be expensive."

"That's okay. I have some money set aside that I can use to pay for it," she said matter-of-factly.

She told me her son Justin lives alone in a house nearby. She explained how Justin's second wife, Cassie, had left him, taking her share of the business. "She bought a motor home and started traveling around with another woman," she laughed.

Poor Justin. His first wife died, then, his second wife left him, with half of her share of the business, and took off with a woman companion. Such a rotten deal!

That evening I took the four tiles that needed cutting to an Ace Hardware store, feeling certain that it would have facilities on hand to cut them. It didn't, but suggested I try a nearby tile store, which is where I had been the day before trying to match up the broken tiles at the back of Maude's bathtub.

I went to the tile store. I was in luck. The man waiting on me said, yes, they could cut the tiles for me, but at one dollar a cut. What a deal! "Do it," I told the man, handing him the four tiles, telling him to cut half an inch off each one.

While I was waiting for the tile to be cut, I selected 14 new tiles for the end of the bathtub. I showed the woman sales clerk one of Maude's tiles and asked her to recommend a solid color that would match. She selected an off-white, saying she thought they would match very well. I needed seven tiles beveled on one side, and one tile beveled on two adjoining sides, and she said she didn't have them in stock, that she would have to order them from a warehouse and I could come back and pick them up on Tuesday. Fine.

The Next Day, Visit 6

I was excited when I arrived at Maude's at 10 a.m. I had the cut tiles with me and could install them on the wall behind the toilet. I was making progress! I parked in Maude's driveway alongside a tan Chevrolet Malibu, which I figured must be owned by Maude's new live-in caregiver for Rusty.

I went in the back door and up the back stairs, calling out my usual "Hello. Maude, it's me, Joe. Hello."

"Come on in," I heard Maude say from the kitchen. She was sitting at the kitchen table reading.

"Hi, Maude," I said, sitting down at the table facing her. "I had those four squares of tile cut and am ready to install them."

"Okay. I hired my live-in caregiver."

"You did?"

"She's in with Rusty now, feeding him."

"That's nice," I told her. "Well, I'm going to get to work and install those four tiles I had cut. I had them take half an inch off each one." I handed her a receipt for four dollars, and she went to her purse and returned with four one-dollar bills.

"Before you start to work, stop in Rusty's bedroom and tell the caregiver what you will be doing."

"Okay."

I went into Rusty's bedroom, where a woman was feeding him breakfast. She was about my height and rather stocky. I guessed her age to be about 60. Her skin color was a light brown, prompting me to conclude she was biracial.

"Hi. My name is Joe, and I'm a hospice volunteer assigned to visit Rusty. I've sort of taken on a bit of a repair job in the bathroom and will be in there installing some ceramic tile. If you want in the bathroom, just holler, and I'll get out of there for you."

"Hi, Joe. My name is Rustylynn. Nice to meet you. I won't be wanting to go into the bathroom for a while. Go ahead and do your repair job."

"You say your name is Rustylynn?"

"Yes, that's right. It's quite a coincidence I should be caring for a man named Rusty. I was named for my father, whose name was Rusty."

"Is that right! That is quite a coincidence."

I went into the bathroom and set about adhesive bonding the four tiles behind the toilet. What a relief! With half an inch cut off each one, they fit perfectly! Then I got to work to bond the six tiles to the wall at the front of the bathtub. Now, if only I had those 14 tiles for the horizontal ledge at the back of the tub.

Just as I was finishing the bonding, Justin entered the bathroom.

"Hi, Justin." I explained how I had to have half an inch removed from the four tiles behind the toilet. I showed them how I bonded the four behind the toilet and the six at the front of the tub. "I'll come back Monday and apply the grout. And I bought fourteen off-white tiles for the ledge at the back of the tub, and I'll come back Tuesday and apply those."

"Okay. It looks nice. You're making good progress," Justin said, approving of what I was doing. "Say, Joe, I wonder if you would help me move a piece of furniture for my mother. We're getting a bedroom fixed up for the caregiver."

"Sure, I'll be happy to."

Justin led me into the bedroom just to the east of the bathroom and had me help him carry a dresser into Maude's bedroom. It was really heavy, but the two of us managed to move it.

"Say, Justin, I've got an idea on how to fix that big open space at the end of the bathroom sink counter. Can I show you my plan?"

We went into the bathroom, and I told Justin how I planned to stuff some wood filler in, let it get hard, and then on Monday fill in the rest of it with some silicone caulk. "Go for it," Justin told me. "Sounds like a good idea."

Justin left, and I got the wood filler out. It was low enough in viscosity to fill in a good share of the open space, which was as wide in places as half an inch. Maude had told me that the guys who had installed that sink counter had done a terrible job. I agreed.

I went into the kitchen and sat down at the table to chat with Maude. Justin was helping Rustylynn carry her packages into the bedroom from where Justin and I moved out the dresser.

"You're bringing in a lot of stuff, aren't you," Maude told Rustylynn.

I was noticing that too. A number of sacks contained groceries, and I saw a big bunch of bananas in one of them.

"I always bring enough provisions to stay for fourteen days," Rustylynn said.

"Maybe you won't have to stay that long,"

Maude said, meaning that Rusty might die before that time.

During one of Justin's and Rustylynn's trips to her car to bring in packages, Maude told me, "She has kinky hair," and laughed. Just as she said this, Justin and Rustylynn entered the kitchen. I had hoped that Rustylynn hadn't heard her.

"How's everything going?" I said loudly to Justin and Rustylynn in order to divert Maude from saying anything more about kinky hair. It worked. I couldn't believe Maude had said that. Was she racially insensitive? I had grown fond of her and hoped I was wrong.

Justin and Rustylynn took some packages into Rustylynn's bedroom, and Maude began to deride Rustylynn. "The nerve of her, wanting to make all those changes to that bedroom. I was using it as a sewing room. She even had Justin move a china closet out of there."

I real quick changed the subject again before Rustylynn returned to the kitchen and picked up the phone. "I'm going to call the hospice and ask for a nurse to come out here and check Rusty's catheter. He's got some bleeding at his penis." She called the hospice and, being unable to reach the nurse at that moment, left word for the nurse to return her call.

"Rusty wants the catheter taken out. And I don't like changing a diaper when a catheter is there," she said. "I changed him earlier this morning and he was really messy. But he ate his breakfast real good."

I looked into Rusty's bedroom several more times, and each time he appeared to be asleep.

"I never did find my hearing aid," Maude said. "Joe, would you mind going into the living room and looking under my chair. Maybe it's under there."

"I would be happy to." I went into the living room and tipped up all sides of the recliner chair and got down on my hands and knees, but saw no traces of her hearing aid.

Back in the kitchen as I was getting ready to go, Rustylynn told Maude, "Did you know you can keep bananas in the refrigerator?"

Something told me I didn't want to hang around to hear Maude's response, lest there be a dispute. I bade farewell to Maude and Rustylynn and left. It was 12:10.

Driving home I suddenly remembered that I hadn't told Maude I had searched under her recliner chair but didn't find her hearing aid. Oh, well. I'll tell her next time I see her.

Two Days Later, Visit 7

I arrived at 9:30 eager to get at the tile repair in Maude's bathroom. I entered the back door, calling out as usual, and receiving no reply and seeing no one in the kitchen, I went into Rusty's bedroom. Maude and Rustylynn were standing by Rusty's bed.

I spoke to Rusty, and he seemed alert. Although he still didn't know who I was, he communicated with me very well. I had him laughing real hard, telling him I was "Joe-Joe from Kokomo, riding on a buffalo." He repeated this for me several times. He looked the best I had seen him so far. His hair was combed and the head of his bed was raised so he was almost sitting up.

I went into the bathroom and grouted the tile I had bonded on Saturday: four squares behind the toilet and six squares in front of the tub. While I had some fresh grout mixed, I looked around the bathroom and added grout wherever it was needed. Then I applied caulk around the edge of the sink counter. The caulk nicely filled in the opening I had partially closed with the wood filler. I stood back and admired my work. The ceramic tile grouting looked great! So did the caulk job around the sink counter! Hey, Joe, you're not too bad as a bathroom repairman! All that remained to be done was to apply the 14 squares of white tile to the ledge at the rear of the tub.

I sat down opposite Maude at the kitchen table. "Will you continue visiting us after you finish repairing the bathroom?"

I laughed. "Well, as a hospice volunteer, I'm supposed to be visiting Rusty. Sure, I'll continue visiting you when I finish with the bathroom."

Back in Rusty's bedroom, I noticed for the first time a Bose radio on a dresser along the wall at the foot of Rusty's bed. I had seen numerous ads for Bose radios, and knew they were very expensive, but I had never seen one. I turned it on and selected 98.7, WFMT, which plays classical music. It was a Mozart sonata. The ads say Bose radios have a unique high-quality sound all of their own. I listened very attentively. It sounded like any other radio to me!

"Do you like this music, Rusty?"

"Yes," he replied decisively. "I don't like the

other music."

Maude had told me that Rustylynn had been playing gospel music for Rusty. "You mean gospel music? You don't like gospel music?"

"No," he said just as decisively.

Rustylynn came into the room. "Rusty said he likes this music, Rustylynn. I tuned in 98.7, WFMT, and they're playing a Mozart sonata."

"Yes, I know."

"You recognized it as a Mozart sonata?"

"Yes, I play the piano and love Mozart," she smiled.

"Someone's in the driveway," Rusty interrupted. He was looking to his left out a window and saw a car pull up.

"It's the Meals on Wheels," I said. A tall, attractive blonde woman of about 40 was carrying two of the meals heading for the back door.

I said good-bye to Rusty and went into the kitchen. Maude was still sitting at the kitchen table. The Meals on Wheels woman set the packaged meals on the kitchen counter. "Be careful, they're very hot," she said, and left.

"Rustylynn has Rusty believing in God," Maude confided.

"Is that right?" I hadn't known Rusty did not believe in God.

"She reads to him a lot from the Bible."

"No kidding! That's wonderful!"

Rustylynn came into the kitchen and handed me a letter. "Will you mail this for me?"

"Sure."

Maude got up and, using her walker, left the kitchen.

"I'm only supposed to care for the patient," she confided, "but I'm doing a lot for Maude, since she can't do much. I'm cooking and doing housecleaning."

"Gee, that's wonderful, Rustylynn! How nice of you! And I suppose it helps time to pass, keeping yourself busy."

I said good-bye to Rustylynn, Maude, and Rusty, and headed for my car. It was 11:15. Out of curiosity I glanced at the front of Rustylynn's letter. It was addressed to a Catholic Church. I guess that means she's a Catholic!

About half way home it suddenly occurred to me I had forgot my toolbox. I must have left it on the floor in the kitchen. When I got home I called Maude's house. Rustylynn answered. "I left my toolbox there," I told her.

"I saw it. I'll set it aside for you."

"Thanks, Rustylynn. I'll be back tomorrow to finish up the bathroom."

In the evening I went to the tile store. They had told me the tile wouldn't be in until Tuesday, but I had a hunch. It was in! I checked each piece. They had it perfect: six squares beveled on one side, one square beveled on two adjoining sides, and seven squares without beveling.

The Next Day, Visit 8

At 9:30 a.m. I parked in the driveway and went in the unlocked back door, calling out, "Maude, hello, it's Joe." Maude was sitting at the kitchen table working a crossword puzzle.

"The hospice nurse and Rustylynn are in with Rusty," she told me. "The nurse is removing Rusty's catheter."

"I was going to get right to work in the bathroom, installing those fourteen new squares of white tile on that bathtub ledge. But I had better wait until the nurse leaves. She may want to use the bathroom." I didn't want to go into Rusty's bedroom while the nurse was with him.

I sat down across the table from Maude, and we chatted. About 15 minutes later the nurse came into the kitchen. It was Peggy, whom I had run into at other hospice patients' houses. She's attractive, cheerful, and always seems glad to see me.

"Hi, Peggy. Good to see you," I smiled, getting up to shake her hand.

"Hi, Joe," she beamed, grasping my hand.

"Isn't Rusty a delight!" I said. "I just love him."

"Isn't he though! He's really something," Peggy replied.

I explained to Peggy how as a hospice volunteer, I elected to do things around the house to help Maude.

"Come into the bathroom, Peggy, and I'll show you what I'm doing."

She followed me, radiant as usual, anxious to see my project. I proudly showed her my tile repair behind the toilet and at the front of the tub, and told her how I came over today to install 14 new squares of tile on the ledge at the back of the bathtub. I showed her how I had caulked around the sink and told her how Maude had asked me to tighten the toilet seat for her.

"Joe, it looks like you're really doing a good job," she smiled. "That's so nice of you, trying to be helpful to Maude."

"Well, with a full-time caregiver, there's not much I can do for Rusty. So I directed my attention at helping Maude instead."

Peggy left, and I went into Rusty's bedroom to talk to him briefly before I went to work in the bathroom. I held his hand and went through my "Joe-Joe from Kokomo" routine. He again had no idea who I was, yet he was able to answer my questions. I tried but failed to get him to laugh.

I managed to bond the white tiles to the bathtub ledge without any problems, being careful to install the tiles with the single beveled sides, the one tile with the two adjoining beveled sides, and the ones without beveled sides in their proper places. There! It looked nice, minus, of course, the grout, which you're not supposed to put on until after at least a few hours to give the adhesive time to set.

I went into the kitchen and told Maude I had bonded the white tile and would come back in the afternoon to grout it. She said she wanted to go out in the yard and check on a few things.

"Would you mind if I accompany you?" I asked.

"Not at all. Come on."

"Can I help you down the back stairs?"

"No," she laughed. "I can get down the stairs just fine. I do it all the time."

She used her walker to get to the top of the stairs and then held onto the railing to go downstairs. "I keep another walker in the garage that I use," she said, using a remote to open one of two doors to the two-car garage.

I got the walker for her out of the garage. Leaning on the walker, she began to stroll about her yard. She picked up a few scraps of paper and an errant stick here and there.

"I can't get over how beautiful the oak trees are in your yard and also in Justin's yard," I told her. "I believe they're bur oaks."

"Is that what they are? I knew they were oaks but I didn't know what kind. Do you know what those two trees are on the west side of the house?" she asked me.

"Yes. They're ash trees," I told her. That is, I was reasonably certain they were ash.

"Very good! That's right. The one on the left is a male, and the one on the right is a female. The female is real dirty, dropping a mess onto the yard every spring."

"Male and female? Is that right!"

We walked along the east side of her house, actually the garage, and I pointed out to her that she had a broken window.

"Yes. It's been broken for a long time. I couldn't seem to get Rusty or Justin to replace it."

"I'll replace it for you. I'll do it for you next Monday. I won't be able to come back until then, because my wife and I have to go to Carbondale tomorrow to visit with her brother."

"You will replace the window?"

"Sure. That's a piece of cake. No problem."

"My goodness. Is there anything you can't

fix?"

I laughed. "Sure. Lots of things. But I'm having pretty good luck so far fixing things around your house."

Maude parked her walker in the garage, and we went up the back stairs into the kitchen. I gave her the receipts for the new tile, the grout, and the adhesive. The bill came to $35, and she gave me a $50 bill. I gave her a $10 bill, which was all I had in my wallet, and told her I would use the $5 to buy glass and putty to replace the broken garage window. She liked that idea.

I left at 11:15 and returned at 3:30 to apply grout around the tiles I had bonded that morning. When I was finished, I couldn't believe how nice it looked. Hey, Joe, it looks like this job was done by a pro!

Back in the kitchen I asked Maude and Rustylynn not to get the newly grouted tile wet until tomorrow. They both went into the bathroom to inspect it and complimented me.

"I know another job you could do," Rustylynn said. "Maude wants a chair in the kitchen that she can scoot around on. Can you put wheels on that chair she sits on at the kitchen table?"

I looked carefully at the chair. "I think I could. But those chair legs are so thin, the casters might break off. That would make it very unsafe for Maude. The best bet would probably be to get her one of those swivel office chairs with casters. I'll look around at a couple of stores and see how much they cost."

I went back into Rusty's room and sat down by his bed and held his hand for a while, again

going through the "Joe-Joe from Kokomo routine."
He communicated with me but again had no idea
who I was.

I left at 4:30, breathing a sigh of joy. I was
finally done with Maude's bathroom! Wow! That
was a tough job. I felt good about the project. Now
Maude's bathroom is as good as new, what with
all the ceramic tile repaired. And didn't that white
tile on the bathtub ledge turn out nice!

Six Days Later, Visit 9

While Dorothy and I were in Carbondale last
Wednesday, Thursday, and Friday, I went into the
Staples store, next to Best Inn where we were
staying, and looked over its line of office chairs
that swivel and ride on casters. They ranged in
simplistic designs from as low as $39 to luxury
models as high as $500 and more.

I was thinking about the office chairs as I
eased my car into Maude's driveway at 11:15 a.m.
I met Maude in the kitchen and told her I was
going to replace her broken garage window. I had
measured it last Tuesday and had acquired a
pane of glass for it on Saturday.

Replacing the broken glass was a piece of
cake. No complications. Many home-repair jobs
run into unexpected problems, as anyone who
has ever done home repairs quickly learns. My
main concern was not to cut myself or get a shard
of glass in my eye. I wore protective glasses to
eliminate that possibility. When I was done, the
completed job looked very professional.

"There, Maude. Your garage broken window is

replaced and is as good as new. What else can I do for you?"

She got up from her kitchen chair and, using her walker, led me into the bathroom.

"You left some caulk on the wall along this edge of the counter," she told me.

"I did? Well, I know how to correct that," I smiled.

Using my fingers, I rubbed off the caulk residue. How careless of me! I glanced at my ceramic tile job. It looked great! I went back in the kitchen, where Maude was again sitting at the table.

"There, Maude. I cleaned up that caulk. Now it's as good as new. Sorry I didn't clean it up earlier. Guess I forgot. Oh, say, I was looking over some office chairs down in Carbondale, and I think I know just the kind to get for you. I think I can get one that you would like for about a hundred dollars. Would you like me to get you one?"

Maude laughed. "That would be nice. Then I could get about my kitchen without getting up. It's always difficult for me to get up and use my walker. Get me a nice one."

"Okay. I'll go over to Office Max this afternoon and get you one."

"Office Max? Why go that far? Can't you get one around here some place?"

"I go to the Office Max store all the time. It's not too far from where I live."

At 1:30 I left home heading for Office Max to buy Maude a chair. I found a nice one originally priced at $129.99 on sale for $99.99. I sat on it and scooted around. It had a high back on it and felt very comfortable. The chair was covered with a dark fabric. It came in a rather large box unassembled. I paid for it and put it in the trunk of my car and headed for Maude's.

I called out "Maude, I'm back," heading up the back stairs entering the kitchen. No one was there, and I went into the hallway, Rustylynn was stretched out on her bed watching TV.

"Hi, Rustylynn. I bought Maude a chair."

"She's taking her nap."

"Oh, okay. I'll go ahead and bring the chair into the kitchen and start assembling it."

At 2:45 I had the chair put together. I sat on it to test it out and scooted about on the linoleum kitchen floor. It felt great, and the casters worked fine. I was sure Maude would like it. Or would she? I had a tinge of a doubt.

I didn't want to leave until Maude tried out the chair, so I stuck my head into her bedroom. She was lying on her left side asleep.

"Maude, I bought you a chair," I said softly.

"You bought me a chair?" she said quickly, and sat up.

As she was standing up and going to her walker, I prayed out loud, for her benefit, "Lord, please let Maude like the chair so I won't have to take it back."

I followed her into the kitchen. As soon as she saw the chair, she said, "I like it. You won't have to take it back."

I felt good watching Maude sit down in the chair and begin to scoot about the kitchen. With some difficulty she began to move herself forward.

"Turn yourself around and scoot yourself backward, Maude, and it will be a lot easier," I told her. She took my advice and was pushing herself around with ease.

"Now I can get around the kitchen without getting out of my chair," she smiled.

I went into Rusty's room and sat down and talked to him for a while. He wasn't very communicative. His Bose radio, with the volume turned down, was still playing classical music on 98.7.

I went back in the kitchen, and Maude wrote me a check for $106.50, the chair's total cost, counting sales tax. I thanked her and left, telling her I would return on Thursday.

Driving home, I thought about the chair. There was something about it I didn't like. What was it? It suddenly hit me! The chair's dark, almost black fabric. It was too somber. I should have picked out one with a bit of color on it, or at least one that wasn't black. Although Maude had said she liked it, somehow, I didn't feel good about the chair.

Three Days Later, Visit 10

I arrived at 11:30 with no particular objective. I had finished repairing the bathroom. I had bought Maude a chair so she could scoot around in her kitchen. I had replaced the broken garage window. Maybe I could visit with Rusty and sit and talk for a while with Maude.

"Maude is sleeping," Rustylynn told me.

I went in to visit with Rusty, but he was pretty much out of it. He didn't look very good and he was totally uncommunicative.

"He almost died yesterday," Rustylynn said.

"He did?"

"Yes. I thought sure he was going to die."

A car pulled into the driveway and a tall middle-aged man entered the kitchen and introduced himself as Rusty's doctor. Rustylynn led him into Rusty's bedroom and awakened Maude to tell her the doctor was here.

Rustylynn returned to the kitchen and told me, "Maude changed her mind about the chair. She doesn't like it and wants you to take it back."

I looked around the kitchen. The chair was gone.

"Where is the chair?" I asked.

"She put it in the hallway. It's at the end of the hallway."

I stuck my head in the hallway and looked. There it was at the end of the hallway in front of the entrance to the end bedroom, the bedroom where Maude told me her daughter and son-in-law from out of state stay occasionally. The chair looked out of place in the hallway. It was so black. And it had such a high back. Why did I ever pick it out for Maude? What was I thinking?

"Oh, by the way," Rustylynn said, "I won't be here next week when you come. My sister Sarah is going to fill in for me. I've been here thirteen days straight, and on Sunday, my fifteenth day, Sarah's coming to take over. I need to get away from here. I like Maude, but she's hard to be with day in and day out. If it weren't for my faith in

God, I would have walked out of here a long time ago. But when I go on a job, I turn everything over to God. And I made an agreement to come here and take care of Rusty. He's my patient. I never break an agreement. But it's God that carries me through."

When Maude came into the kitchen, I told her I was going home to get my tools and would be back to take apart the chair and return it to Office Max. She seemed pleased.

"I liked the chair at first," she said, "but then it began to hurt my legs." She pointed to the upper part of her legs. "I don't want to sit in a chair that hurts my legs."

"I don't blame you, Maude. I wouldn't want to sit in a chair that hurt my legs either."

"Another thing I didn't like about that chair was I couldn't scoot into the hallway."

I glanced toward the hallway. No wonder. The hallway is carpeted!

"To scoot into the hallway, you would need something with bigger wheels," I told her.

I returned to Maude's house at 1:30 and wrote her a check for $107 for the chair. I then disassembled it.

"Maude, would you like to come with me to Office Max and pick out a chair?"

"No. Just forget it. I'll just sit in my chair like I always do."

Justin came up the back stairs into the kitchen and helped me carry the chair out to my car. I told Maude I would return on Monday.

At Office Max they took back the chair

without any problem. The chair episode was now history. Oh, well, I tried to please her. But that big black chair *was* ugly.

Four Days Later, Visit 11

At 11 a.m., Rustylynn's sister Sarah was in the kitchen. I introduced myself and started chatting with her. She said Maude was sitting in the living room reading. She told me a bit about her and Rustylynn's family back in Texas, where she said her parents had 200 acres. She confided that her father was white and her mother was black. Sarah had light-brown skin like Rustylynn. She was stocky like Rustylynn but perhaps slightly shorter and maybe not as heavy. Just as I liked Rustylynn, I took an immediate liking to Sarah.

While I was talking with her, the Meals on Wheels car came. I went out to the driveway and carried in the meals, being warned by the driver not to burn myself because the plates were very hot, which indeed they were.

I went into Rusty's bedroom to visit with him. He seemed to be in a trance, totally uncommunicative, so I left him and went into the living room to chat with Maude. She talked about her children and grandchildren, pointing to pictures on the wall.

I left at noon.

Two Days Later, Visit 12

I had been thinking about Maude and her desire to have a chair with wheels on which she could scoot around. It had become apparent that an office chair with regular-sized casters was no good because the chair would not move across the hallway carpeting. What she needed, I concluded, was a chair with wheels of perhaps four inches or more in diameter.

A few days earlier I had received in the mail Dr. Leonard's catalog of various health-care items, including some elder-care chairs with large wheels. I left my house at about 9:15 a.m., bringing along the Dr. Leonard's catalog. I stopped at a hospital supply store and inquired about chairs with large wheels. I was shown several different styles and was given a few brochures.

When I got to Maude's house, I showed her the Dr. Leonard's catalog and the hospital supply store flyers. She said she did not want any of the chairs shown in either the catalog or the flyers. She said to just forget about it, and she would be content to sit in her kitchen chair, one without wheels.

"Okay, Maude. I'll just forget about it. But it was fun trying to help you come up with a chair with wheels of your liking."

"Say, I've got something else for you to fix, if you want," she smiled.

"What do you have in mind?"

"My kitchen faucet leaks." She took me over to the sink. When she turned on the faucet, water leaked from around the bottom of the faucet.

"I think I can fix it," I told her. I examined the faucet and found the make: Moen.

"I'm pretty sure I can get a repair kit for it," I

told her. "I'll stop at Ace Hardware on the way home and check it out."

I studied her faucet again, noting that the plumbing under the kitchen sink did not have a shut-off valve for either the hot or cold water. "If I have to do repairs on the faucet, I'll probably have to turn the water off coming into the house."

"That would be all right, providing you don't have it turned off for very long," Maude said.

"In case I should have to replace the faucet, I would recommend installing shut-off valves under the sink. But let's not talk about that until I see if I can repair the faucet with a kit."

I decided to do a little exploratory "probing" on the faucet. I went out to my car and brought in a few tools and was able to remove the faucet's movable spigot without turning off the house water. I spotted a couple of O-rings that probably needed to be replaced. I took them off and traced out their size on a piece of paper. Then I put the faucet back together. I turned the water on.

"Guess what, Maude. The faucet doesn't leak anymore. My taking it apart and putting it back together fixed the leak," I laughed. "But I'll try to buy the repair kit. I don't think the leak will stay fixed for very long."

Before I left, I went in to look at Rusty. Sarah was with him, and Rusty appeared to be in a trance. I wondered if he was in the initial stages of dying. I didn't even try to communicate with him.

On the way home I stopped at an Ace Hardware. It didn't have the repair kit I needed and recommended I try a nearby specialty plumbing shop.

I went to the shop and, sure enough, they had the kit. I compared the O-rings in the kit to those I had traced on a piece of paper from Maude's faucet. They were the exact size I needed!

Two Days Later, Visit 13

I arrived at Maude's at 2:45 and repaired her kitchen faucet by replacing the two O-rings. The leak was gone! All I charged Maude was $3.15 that the shop charged me for the kit. While Maude was getting money out of her purse to reimburse me, Justin came into the kitchen. I told him what I did to repair the sink faucet.

"I was worried I might have to replace the faucet," I told him. "But the repair kit solved the problem just fine!"

I went in to see Rusty again, and Sarah told me that Rusty, still in a trance-like stupor, is beginning to talk to spirits.

"He is?"

"Yes. I've seen a lot of people die, and shortly before they pass, they all begin talking to spirits."

"Is that right?"

She assured me it was indeed right.

Sarah asked me how old Rusty was, and I told her 93.

I left at 3:50.

The Next Day, Visit 14

I parked my car in Maude's driveway at 2:30 and went in the back door and up the stairs to the kitchen, calling out softly, "Hello, it's Joe." The kitchen was empty, and I went into the hallway and into Rusty's bedroom. The two beds had been switched. The double bed was now near the windows, and Rusty and his hospital bed were near the hallway. The head of Rusty's bed was raised, and Sarah was sitting in a chair on his right feeding him applesauce.

"Hi, Sarah. Hey, I see you've switched the beds around. I guess to get Rusty away from the windows, huh?"

"Yes. The weather got kind of cold, and we thought he would be warmer away from the windows."

"How is he doing? Is he eating the applesauce?"

"He's not doing very well. But he's eating the applesauce pretty good. Shortly before they die, I start giving them mushy stuff like applesauce."

"Is that right? Something easy for them to swallow, I guess, huh? Is Maude taking a nap?"

"No, she's in the living room. I think she's watching TV."

Rusty began to cough. It was a weak cough. He appeared to be in a trance. His eyes were half shut and staring into space. Sarah placed her left hand behind his head to tilt his head forward.

"I do this to help him cough," Sarah said.

Rusty's mouth was drawn. "Did you remove his teeth?" I asked.

"Yes. Shortly before they die, their teeth will often slip and get sideways and such. They're a lot more comfortable with their teeth out."

"I figured he didn't have his teeth in. His mouth looked sort of puckered, as though he had aged considerably since I last saw him."

I glanced about the room. The "lift" that had been used to help get Rusty out of bed was in a corner by a window. A suction device was on a table to Sarah's left. The Bose radio was playing softly and was again tuned to 98.7's classical music.

Something prompted me to peel back the fingers of Rusty's left hand and grasp and hold it. I gently massaged his hand as I held it with both of mine. I began to feel such a peace. Rusty stopped coughing, and Sarah let his head go back on his pillow but kept her left hand behind his head.

"I think he must have had a stroke. His right hand is swollen." Then she started talking softly to Rusty, slowly peeling back each finger. "One, two, three, four. I'm counting your fingers, hon. Did you have a stroke? And did it leave your right hand swollen?"

She pulled her hand from behind his head and caressed his forehead and ran her fingers through his hair.

My spirit drank in the peaceful ambience: A dying old man. A loving caregiver.

"You were telling me the other day that shortly before people die they begin to see spirits, probably the spirits of their loved ones."

"Yes. That's true. I've seen many people die, and they all begin to see the spirits of their loved ones."

She smiled compassionately at Rusty. "Can

you see your mother, hon?" I turned to look at the foot of the bed, half expecting to see his mother. "Is she waiting for you? You can go to her if you want. That's all right. You can go to her, hon."

I continued to massage Rusty's left hand. It felt warm, as though there still remained a lot of life in it. I felt a tear glide down my left cheek. Was I experiencing the joy of death? Was that an oxymoron? Could death be joyful? The peace in the room filled the very fiber of my being. How could this be? It had to be! The joy of death! I had never felt such peace.

I looked ahead in my own life to when I am dying. Oh, how I hope I can have a loving caregiver like Sarah at my bedside. I wanted to tell this to Sarah, but it was as though I couldn't speak. I didn't want the sound of my voice to shatter the peace and love in the room.

After what seemed like many minutes of silence, I asked Sarah, "I think you told me your husband died in January?"

"Yes. He was sixty-four years old." Her left hand continued to caress Rusty's forehead.

"My goodness, but he was still a relatively young man. What did he die of?"

"Of diabetes complications."

Both Sarah and her sister Rustylynn had told me their father was white and their mother was black. I found myself asking Sarah, "Was your husband black?"

"Yes."

"Was he a big man?"

Sarah laughed. "Yes, he was *big* and *macho*!"

"How tall was he?"

"He was six foot five."

"Oh, my goodness! He *was* big and *macho*, wasn't he?"

"He sure was. He was *all* man, if you know what I mean," she laughed.

I thought suddenly of Maude. She apparently was still in the living room.

"Sarah, I had better go in and talk to Maude." I peeled back Rusty's fingers, releasing my right hand. "What a joy it was sitting in here with you and Rusty. I think I was actually experiencing the joy of dying. I hope I have a caregiver like you when I die."

In the living room Maude was sitting in her corner recliner watching TV's Dr. Laura field questions related to love and sex. I couldn't believe it. What was Maude, all of 87 years old, doing watching Dr. Laura?

"Hi, Maude."

"Hi. You came back again."

"Can I watch Dr. Laura with you?"

She laughed. "Sure." She appeared to be hanging onto every word of advice uttered by Dr. Laura.

I sat down in the chair on her left and turned to watch the TV. I had heard Dr. Laura on radio but had never seen her on TV. On radio she seemed so much more livelier, so uninhibited. On TV she seemed wooden and self-conscious. I found myself not listening to what she was saying but wondering why she was so good on radio but lacking in appeal on TV.

"Her program almost went off the air not so long ago. But she's doing better now," Maude said.

"Dr. Laura talks so fast I can hardly understand her. Can you understand her?" Maude asked.

"She does talk fast, doesn't she. I can understand her, but I think I could understand her better if she spoke a bit slower." I tried to frame my reply diplomatically.

When the Dr. Laura program ended, Maude picked up her remote control and turned off the TV. I began asking her about the family pictures on the wall in the living room and hallway.

"I keep *my* family pictures in the hallway, and *Rusty's* family pictures in the living room," Maude smiled. "I also keep our own family pictures in the living room."

I asked Maude about a picture in the hallway of a little girl I thought resembled Maude.

"That's my mother. She was born in 1887, and that picture was taken a long time ago."

"Gee, what a beautiful picture."

Maude identified other hallway pictures as being of her parents and of her brother.

I asked her about a picture of a young woman that looked much like Maude.

"That's me," she smiled, "when I was about twenty."

"You were beautiful! In the picture you look so very Scandinavian."

One picture was of her son Justin and his family. Justin's first wife died of cancer, and a son died of a seizure.

Another picture was of Maude and Rusty and their children when Justin was 11, Janet 9, Richard 7, and Charlotte 1. "What a beautiful family! And look at what a handsome boy Richard was!"

We started talking about Rusty. "It seems that every time Rusty takes a turn for the worse and it appears he is going to die, he always begins to improve. Rusty is stubborn and doesn't want to die," Maude said.

"Well, I think I'll go check on Rusty again," I told her, and left the living room and went into Rusty's bedroom. Sarah was still comforting him, holding his right hand and caressing his head with her left hand. I went around to the other side of Rusty's bed and took Rusty's left hand again.

"I'm waiting for the nurse to come," Sarah said.

"If Rusty should die while I'm not here, would you give me a call, Sarah?"

"Certainly." I wrote down my name and phone number and gave it to her.

I began to think about Sarah having a white father and a black mother.

"You told me you had a white father and a black mother. Do you feel white or do you feel black?" I felt a bit guilty for asking her this.

"I feel neither," she said without hesitation. "I just feel like I'm myself. I don't feel white and I don't feel black. I'm just me," she smiled.

"That's really interesting. You don't feel white or black; you just feel like yourself."

"That's right. Neither white nor black."

"Was Rustylynn's husband black?"

"Yes."

"When did he die?"

"About five years ago."

"I just love the tender loving care you're giving to Rusty. Do you feel such loving care helps prepare the dying for death?"

"Yes, I really do. I think it comforts them and helps put them at peace."

I left Sarah and Rusty and went into the kitchen, where Maude was now sitting in her chair at the table.

"How is that kitchen faucet doing, Maude? Has it started leaking again?"

"No. Not that I know of. But you might go over there and test it and see for yourself."

I went to the faucet, turned it on, and watched for signs of a leak. "Hurrah! It isn't leaking, Maude!"

I sat down across the table from Maude.

"Which funeral home will Rusty be taken to when he dies?" I asked.

She named the funeral home and gave me directions to it.

"I think you said he will be buried in your family plot?"

"Yes. Justin's wife, Harriet, is buried there, and so is his son."

Maude paused and then asked me, "When Rusty dies, will you stop coming?" I recalled that she had asked me that once before. I couldn't remember what I had told her.

"Yes." My reply had such a tone of finality. "Yes, when a patient dies, I'm generally assigned another patient fairly soon, and begin to visit my new patient. But if there's ever anything I can do for you, please don't hesitate to call. I've given you my phone number."

I got up to leave. "Well, Maude, I'm going to shove off now. I'll be back on Thursday. On Tuesday and Wednesday I have to sit with an Alzheimer's patient whom I've been sort of caring for now for over a year."

I got in my car and glanced at my watch. It was 4:15.

Three Days Later, Visit 15

The hospice office called at 1:30 to tell me about a development with Maude. Rusty's caregiver, Sarah, had called the office to report that Maude had insulted her, telling Sarah something like, "You seem to be trying to act like you're white." Sarah said she became so incensed she immediately called her sister Rustylynn to come over as fast as she could to relieve her, or else she was going to walk out on Maude.

With this incident in mind, I headed for Maude's at 2:45. The temperature was in the low 70's as I parked in her driveway. Countless leaves from Maude's ash trees were riding a brisk breeze across the intersection.

I went up the back stairs and into the kitchen calling out my usual, "Hello, it's Joe." I went into the hallway and, glancing to my left, saw

Rustylynn stretched out on her bed watching TV.

"Hi, Rustylynn. It's good to see you again," I told her. She got up and accompanied me into Rusty's bedroom. He was lying on his right side asleep.

"I'm about to switch him to his left side. I like to move my patients from side to side to prevent their getting pneumonia. It's always the pneumonia that kills them. They begin aspirating."

"Where is Maude?" I asked.

"She's in the living room watching TV."

"The hospice office called and told me Maude had insulted Sarah and how Sarah had called you to relieve her or else she was going to walk out."

"I don't let Maude bother me. I don't let anything bother me, because I've turned my life over to God. I'm here to take care of Rusty. Maude can do whatever she wants. After all, it's her house."

"My goodness, but you are certainly filled with wisdom! Wow!" I told her. We turned to look at Rusty, breathing evenly as he slept.

"I had talked with Sarah about her background, and yours, too, having a white father and a black mother, with ten children, and whether she felt white or black. Sarah told me she doesn't feel either white or black, that she just feels like herself."

"That's how I feel, too. Neither white nor black. I just feel like myself."

"Sarah said she had a black husband. Was your husband black, too?"

"Yes."

"I better go in the living room and talk to Maude," I told Rustylynn.

Maude had just turned off the TV and was getting up from her chair.

"I'm hungry," she said, grasping her walker. I followed her past Rusty's bedroom and into the kitchen.

I sat down at the kitchen table as Maude set about warming up a tray of food from Meals on Wheels. She brought it to the table and sat down to eat.

"Well, what else do you have that I can fix?" I smiled.

"Do you know anything about storm windows?"

"Yeah. Why, what's the problem?"

She turned to her right and pointed to the window by her side. "The upper storm window seems to be off its track. I can't budge it. Can you figure out how to get it back on track so I can lower it?"

"Well, let me take a look."

I stood up and looked at the stuck window. I couldn't figure it out. I got up on a kitchen chair and studied it some more. I still couldn't make sense out of it. I went outside to look at the windows. I couldn't believe what I was seeing. The window by the sink, the two windows by Maude's kitchen table, and the two windows by Rusty's bedroom all appeared to have their upper window jammed—installed improperly. In addition, two of the windows by Maude's table had little broken areas in one corner. I studied the windows from outside but I still couldn't figure out how to get them back on track. I went back inside.

"Maude, the only thing I can suggest is to let me bring my tools over tomorrow and start taking apart the windows and see what I can come up with," I told her.

"No, you're not taking them apart," Maude said sternly. "Go over to the business and get Justin. He knows how to fix them."

"It's kind of late to be starting them now. I tell you what. I'll come back tomorrow morning and go over and get Justin and ask him to show me how to fix them. How would that be?"

"Okay," Maude said.

"It looks as if the windows weren't put back properly. Who was the last person to put the windows back in place?"

"The painters. I had some painters here last summer painting the window frames."

"Boy, they sure did a bad job reinstalling the windows, didn't they?"

"Yes," she said. "I've raised and lowered those windows countless times and never had any problem with them. But they're sure jammed now."

We chatted for a few minutes more and then I left. It was 4:10. Driving home I had mixed feelings about those windows. I would love to start taking them apart to try to figure out how they work, but I had to do it Maude's way: get Justin and ask him to show me how to do it.

The Next Day, Visit 16

I eased my car to a stop in Maude's driveway at 9:30 a.m. The weather was clear, and the temperature was about 65. Planes were taking off toward the southwest thundering over the vicinity of Maude's house. I encountered Rustylynn in the kitchen.

"Hi, Rustylynn. Where's Maude?"

"She's in the living room. I've about had it with her!" she told me in all seriousness. "She is so bossy and rude!"

Was this the same Rustylynn who had told me just the day before that she doesn't let Maude affect her because she turns everything over to God? What had happened? Had Maude been extra rude? Had Rustylynn forgot to turn everything over to God?

I went into the living room and told Maude, sitting in her recliner chair reading, I was going over to the business and ask Justin to come over and show me how the storm windows work so I could set about unjamming them. Maude approved, and I went out the back door and headed for the business.

I walked along the side of the garage where I had replaced the broken window. I hadn't been inside the business and wasn't exactly sure where the office was, where I expected to find Justin. I sort of followed my instinct and found myself inside a large area where two women, a blonde and a brunette, were working behind a table.

"Can we help you with something?" the blonde asked. A few weeks ago when I was replacing the garage window I had seen her walking across Justin's yard heading for his house. And a week or so ago she came into Maude's house looking for Justin.

"I'm a hospice volunteer visiting Rusty and helping Maude do some things around the house. She asked me to come over here and get Justin to show me how her storm windows work." Then something made me add, "Maude seems to be in a bad mood this morning."

"*This* morning?" the blonde said, and the brunette laughed.

Justin came out of a nearby office.

"Your mother wonders if you could take a few minutes to come over to the house and show me how those storm windows work. Some of them have been put back improperly, and they seem to be jammed."

"Sure," Justin said. I followed him to the house and up the back stairs into the kitchen. Maude was sitting at the kitchen table.

Justin pulled a chair to the window on Maude's right and stood up on it. He lowered the inner top window and began tugging on the jammed upper storm window.

"Is there anything I can do?" I asked.

"No. This window was put back wrong. I just have to pull on it and hopefully get it to come out."

"Maybe I should get my screwdriver and start taking apart the window assembly from the outside," I volunteered.

"You might well have to do that, but hold off for a few minutes until I see if I can get this window out this way."

He tugged and pulled on the window. I reached up and tried to help him. Finally he started making progress. The window was coming out.

"There, it's coming," Justin said. "Here it comes!" He carefully nudged the window out and set it on the floor against a wall.

"Okay, Justin. I get the idea. I'll use the same procedure to remove the jammed windows on these other windows in the kitchen and the two in Rusty's room."

"Okay," Justin said, and turned and left the kitchen and headed back to his business.

"Well, Maude, now that I've seen Justin do it, I've got my work cut out for me," I laughed. I stood up on the chair and tugged at the jammed window in the next window assembly. Following the same procedure used by Justin, I soon had it out. Then I went to the window over the sink and extracted that jammed window.

With the jammed windows out, it was an easy matter to remove the other two windows and the screen from each window assembly.

"Maude, can I wash these windows for you?"

"Sure," she smiled.

"Do you have some Windex spray?"

"It's under the kitchen sink."

Minutes later I was washing all of the kitchen windows and putting them back in place, except for the two that had broken glass.

"Can I drop off these two broken ones at Ace Hardware for you and get them repaired?"

"Okay. And then I can reimburse you."

In removing the windows and screens, I readily saw how the windows were supposed to be assembled.

"Boy, those painters sure did put these windows back in place the wrong way, didn't they?" I said to Maude.

"I guess they did. I know *I* didn't put them back like that."

"Rustylynn told me you were getting ready to go to a doctor's office for an appointment. Is Justin taking you?" I asked.

"No, I'm taking a cab. I have a cab coming at 10:30."

"You're taking a cab? I could drive you. Why don't you call the cab company and cancel the cab," I suggested.

"No, that's all right. I'll go ahead and take a cab."

"Are you sure? I would love to drive you."

"No, I'll take the cab."

I gave up.

At 10:30 the cab hadn't arrived yet, and Maude was getting antsy. By 10:40 she was about ready to ask me to take her when the cab pulled into her driveway.

The cab driver appeared to be of a Mediterranean nationality. I asked him if he could find her doctor's office, and he said he could.

Continuing to work on the windows, I saw the Meals on Wheels car pull into the driveway at 11 o'clock. I left at 11:20, taking the two broken windows with me. I dropped them off at an Ace

Hardware store to be repaired. The attendant told me they would be ready in about a week.

I returned at 1:45. Rustylynn was in the kitchen, Peggy, the hospice nurse, was in with Rusty, and Maude was in the living room sitting in her recliner reading.

"I've about had it with that woman," Rustylynn told me. "She's really got me upset, and I'm just about ready to walk out," she confided.

I went into the living room to check in with Maude. "Do you think you could re-attach that electrical outlet to the wall by the kitchen stove? Rustylynn or Sarah pulled it off the wall. They just grabbed the electrical plug and yanked on it. I told them they should pull the plug with one hand and hold the outlet with the other so as not to jerk it off the wall. But they didn't listen to me."

"I'll take a look at it," I told her, and headed for the kitchen. I looked at the electrical outlet and where it had been pulled from the wall and decided it needed some longer screws. I went back into the living room to ask Maude if she had any long screws.

"Look in those drawers in the pantry. I think there are some in there," she said.

I found the drawers and three long screws and set about to reattach the electrical outlet to the wall. Rustylynn, watching me, said, "You're going to need some anchor bolts for that. I watched my daddy do a lot of repairs like that, and he always used anchor bolts."

"You're a hundred percent right. If these long screws don't do the trick, I'll go pick up some anchor bolts."

But the long screws worked! I didn't have to get the anchor bolts after all.

Peggy had left Rusty's room and went in the living room to talk with Maude. I went into Rusty's room to start working to unjam the windows that had been mounted improperly. Peggy returned to the room, and we exchanged greetings.

"How's Rusty doing?" I asked her.

"I've told Rustylynn to stop feeding him and to discontinue giving him drinks."

I couldn't believe what I had just heard. That sounded to me like the sentence of death for Rusty. No food? No water?

"Rustylynn told me she was up this morning from three o'clock on with Rusty because he kept choking. He can no longer swallow without choking. When that happens, it's no use to try to get them to eat or drink anymore," she explained. "I told Rustylynn to use a little sponge to moisten his mouth periodically." Peggy showed me the sponge that she had set out for Rustylynn. It was a petite-looking little cube attached to a stick-like holder.

Peggy left and Rustylynn came into Rusty's bedroom and began to tell me again how she was about ready to walk out.

"Rustylynn, why don't you get in your car and go some place and calm down. Go to a park and take a walk, or go to a store and do some shopping, anything to get away from this house for a while. I'll be here to tend to Rusty if he needs anything," I told her.

"That's a good idea," she said. "I'll tell Maude I need to go to the store."

Within minutes Rustylynn left, and I began working on the windows in Rusty's room. I pulled out the jammed window from the top of each of the window assemblies, then set about taking out the windows and screens and washing them. At Maude's suggestion, I left a screen in the down position in one of the windows to permit fresh air to enter the room.

I asked Maude if I could mount storm windows on the front and back doors for her, and with her approval, I quickly had that done, washing the windows on each door. I put the door screens in Maude's basement.

I decided to walk around the house and see if anymore storm windows appeared to be jammed. They all looked satisfactory except for the two window assemblies on the south side of the southeast bedroom, the room that Maude said she uses for guests. These windows appeared to be hopelessly jammed and abandoned by someone, probably the painters.

Returning into the house, I saw Maude sitting at the kitchen table eating a Meal on Wheels dinner she had heated. What was this she was eating? It looked like fried shrimp! Not just one or two, but at least half a dozen or more. They looked delicious.

"Would you like one?" she asked.

"No thanks. Boy, look at all those shrimps! Is that a Meal on Wheels?"

"Yes," she laughed. "I took Rusty's shrimps, because he won't be eating them. You sure you won't have one?"

"No thanks."

"I just can't give you anything, can I?" she smiled. "You know, I've never met anyone like you before."

I changed the subject. "I found a couple more jammed windows—on that bedroom on the southeast corner of the house. I'll come back Monday and fix those for you," I told her.

"Okay." She took a bite of shrimp and said, "I think I've been nagging Rustylynn too much. I've hurt her feelings. I have to stop that."

I wanted to say something, yet held back. So, she *had* been aware of her nagging!

Then she started telling me about her children: Janet lives about 60 miles away with her husband, who is a twin. Charlotte lives in another state with her husband, who is also a twin. Charlotte and her husband both perform in an orchestra.

She told me she has a lawn service cut her grass and rake her leaves. I looked out the window, and a brisk breeze was blowing leaves from Maude's ash trees across the intersection.

While I was walking around her house, I happened to notice that the house has what appears to be a large attic. I asked Maude about it.

"Would you like to go up there and take a look?" she asked.

"Sure. How do I get up there?"

"Through the door at the end of the hallway."

"Okay, I'll go up and look around."

I opened the door and walked up the steep stairway. There was no railing. The attic smelled musty, as though no one had been up there for years. There was a lot of dust and cobwebs. But I couldn't get over how much room there was. After a quick inspection, I went back down the stairs to Maude at the kitchen table.

"That is really a big attic," I told her.

"I might have it fixed up for my family for when they visit. With Rusty ill and near death, I can do that now. I can do whatever I want without Rusty objecting."

It was almost 4:30 and I was beginning to get anxious for Rustylynn to return. Where was she? I had promised her I would stay until she got back.

"Would you like me to go in and sponge Rusty's mouth for him?" I asked Maude. I was hoping she would say no, because I had never sponged a dying person's mouth. In fact, I had never sponged anyone's mouth.

"You better not. Rustylynn might get upset. She might think I told you to do it because I was afraid she might not do it right."

"Okay."

I went in to look at Rusty. He was semicomatose. His left ear appeared to be swollen. I had asked Peggy about this, and she said they get that way shortly before death. The Bose radio was still playing classical music on 98.7. It sounded like another Mozart piano sonata.

I went back into the kitchen. I picked up a pair of pliers Justin had left on the table when he was working on the window. "Can I put these away for you, Maude?"

"Yes. They go in that drawer over by the sink. Justin and Rusty are just like Rusty's father. They never put things back where they found them."

Then she changed the subject. "You know, Rusty and I used to sit at this table a lot. I would sit here, and Rusty would sit where you're sitting. I would tell him what I was seeing over there at the corner to the west, and he would tell me what he was seeing down the street to the east."

"That is so sweet," I smiled. "I wonder when Rustylynn is going to come back."

"You can leave if you want."

"No, I promised Rustylynn I would stay until she returned. And a promise is a promise."

"Here she comes," Maude said.

I looked out the window as Rustylynn's car turned into the driveway. I breathed a sigh of joy.

Seconds later Rustylynn entered the kitchen.

"Oh, my goodness, I thought I'd never get back. Traffic was a nightmare—a parking lot!"

"Yeah, traffic really gets heavy around here at this time of day. Well, guess I'll go now." I glanced at my watch. It was 4:40.

Three Days Later, Visit 17

At 11:30 I played a message on our phone recorder. It was the hospice office telling me Rusty died at about 3 o'clock yesterday afternoon. I was saddened, as I had told Maude I would return Monday afternoon and fix and clean the south windows in the southeast bedroom. Also, I had told Rustylynn I would fill in for her on Wednesday.

Even though Rusty had died, I arrived at the house at 1:45. A car was parked on the street, but no cars were in the driveway. I sort of expected family members from out of town to be there. I went in the back door and loudly said, "Hello."

A young voice answered, "Hello, come on in."

I went into the kitchen and Maude was sitting at the table, and a young lady was standing talking to her. She introduced herself to me as Hattie, Janet's daughter, and said she works at a nearby firm as an assistant manager. She was attractive, with blue eyes and blonde hair. I sat down at the table opposite Maude.

I told them I had heard that Rusty had died, that I had promised Maude I would come Monday and fix those two windows for her, "that a promise is a promise." Hattie said Maude had spoken highly of me. The kitchen seemed very warm. Within minutes I excused myself to get to work on the windows, with Maude's permission, of course.

Justin came in the room as I was getting started, and I told him how easy it was to work on those windows now that I knew how to do it. Justin told me about Rusty's dying, how he, Janet, and Rustylynn were with him when he died, but that Maude was in the living room. Justin said as soon as he died, Rustylynn got ready to leave and said she couldn't wait to get into her own house and soak in her own bathtub.

Within about 20 minutes, I reassembled the windows and washed them.

I went into the kitchen and sat down across from Maude again. She was working a crossword puzzle. Maude said she and Justin went this morning to select a suit of clothes and a coffin for Rusty. Justin was going to prepare a large basket of flowers for the casket. I wrote down when the wake was going to be and told Maude I'd be there.

She read me the obituary she had prepared for the newspaper.

On the way home I remembered I had forgot to wash the inside surfaces of the inside windows. I stopped at the Ace Hardware store; Maude's windows were ready, but I didn't have the receipt with me, so I didn't pick them up. I had misunderstood the man when I left them. I thought he had said a man would come and pick up the broken windows, repair them, and bring them back to the store, and the whole process would take about a week. But what he had meant was that a guy comes once a week and repairs the windows right in the store. The name the clerk wrote on the windows was misspelled, but I recognized my phone number. I decided to pick them up Wednesday and take them to Maude's house.

The Next Day

I found Rusty's obituary in this morning's newspaper. I made plans to attend the wake this evening.

I arrived at the funeral home at 6:10 and readily found the designated parlor. I went in and saw a sparse scattering of people standing around talking. I made my way slowly up front toward the brown casket. I was looking for Maude but didn't see her. I went up to Justin, who was talking with several people. He recognized me and shook my hand and thanked me for coming. I turned and went to the casket and looked down at Rusty. He resembled a distinguished, retired businessman taking a siesta after a hard day at the office. His gray hair was meticulously combed. His mouth was full, as though he had his teeth in. The makeup on his facial skin made him look alive. He was handsome in his brown suit, white shirt, and tie.

Rusty, it was nice knowing you. I was so glad I met you while you could still talk and communicate. How good it was to see and hear you laugh when I joked with you about my being Joe-Joe from Kokomo, riding on a buffalo. Thank you, dear God, for creating Rusty, and for giving him a long life.

I turned to speak with Justin and waited a few minutes until he finished talking with some friends.

"Justin, I don't see Maude," I told him.

"She's sitting down in the next room. Let me get her for you." He headed for a door on the north side of the parlor. I followed him slowly, keeping some distance from him, not wanting to go in the room and interrupt Maude. I stopped and waited by the door, turning to avoid looking into the room. Maude, leaning on her walker, came out and spoke to me.

"Hi, Maude. How are you doing?"

"Just fine," she smiled. "I'm glad you came."

"Let's go up and look at Rusty," I suggested.

I walked alongside her as she used her walker. We stopped in front of the casket. She looked down at him compassionately.

"Rusty, I wish you could get up and see everything—see how pretty all the flowers are and see your family and friends," she said softly. I felt my eyes cloud up.

"Doesn't he look good. Just like he's asleep," she said. "It's too bad there aren't more people here. But then I guess Rusty outlived all of his friends."

"Did Justin make up the flower arrangements?" I asked.

"Yes, most of them anyway."

She led me past the floral displays. Stopping at one, she admired what she called "snapdragons."

"Come on, I would like you to meet Richard."

She led me across the parlor to a man standing talking with another man.

"Joe, this is my son, Richard. Richard, this is Joe. He's a hospice volunteer who has been visiting Rusty and was nice enough to fix a number of things around the house."

"Hi, Richard."

We shook hands. He was about my height and had a portly stomach. He was wearing rimmed glasses, and I thought he looked a lot like Rusty. I was impressed with his gentle spirit. Remembering that Maude had told me Richard was autistic, I couldn't discern anything unusual about him. His gentle spirit didn't seem that unusual. He told me he works as a custodian at a store in a nearby suburb.

Maude left us to talk with someone else. Richard took me across the parlor to meet a man and woman sitting down.

"This is Henry and Mae. I live with them," Richard said. They appeared to be perhaps in their 50's. Judging from our conversation, I assumed Richard boarded at their house. They had a serious air of compassion about them, as though they genuinely liked Richard and were interested in his well-being.

I left Richard and made my way back to Maude. She introduced me to her daughters, Janet and Charlotte. Janet had light hair and told me she lives on the shore of a river. She said her husband had always wanted to live on a waterway. I found Janet to be charming, and I liked her immediately.

Charlotte had dark hair and told me she lives in an adjoining state. Although she was nice and friendly, she didn't exude Janet's warmth.

Maude took me around and introduced me to Janet's daughter, Hattie, and to her boyfriend, Pat. I had met Hattie the day before at Maude's house. Then she introduced me to Janet's son, Mark, whom I thought was handsome and self-confident.

I got to talking with Justin again and asked him to show me his floral displays. His eight displays featured red carnations, white roses, and delphiniums. I specifically asked Justin about the flowers Maude referred to as snapdragons, and Justin said they were delphiniums.

I went to the back of the parlor and began studying the large displays of family pictures, many of which showed Rusty. One picture in particular fascinated me. It showed Maude standing next to Rusty, with Maude appearing to be several inches taller. I asked Maude about the picture and how much taller she was than Rusty.

"Rusty was five-six, and I am five seven and a half. The reason I look so much taller than Rusty in that picture is because I was wearing high heels," she laughed.

Also in the back of the room was a big computerized display of the family tree that someone had printed up. I started to study it, but became confused and gave up.

I began speaking to Maude about Richard. "I bet Richard has always been your favorite, hasn't he?" I had visions of Richard being a "momma's boy."

"No, I don't have any favorites. But if I were to have one, it would be Janet. Janet and I get along real well, and we actually like each other."

"I'll be returning your windows on Thursday," I told Maude. "I checked with the Ace Hardware store, and they said they're ready."

"That will be fine," she said.

I went to a table to pick up a remembrance card for Rusty and ran into the two ladies I had met at the business. They introduced themselves as Ellen and Lucy. Ellen was the blonde, and Lucy, the brunette. They said they had worked at the business for 14 years. I briefly alluded to Maude's strong personality, and they said she clashes with almost everyone.

As I was getting ready to leave, I said good-bye to Maude. "You're welcome to come to lunch with us tomorrow after the funeral. It's going to be at that steak house near our house."

"Thanks, Maude, but I think I'll pass on that."

"I just can't get you to accept anything, can I," she smiled.

On the way to my car I ran into Hattie and her boyfriend standing in front of the funeral home smoking cigarettes.

One side of Rusty's remembrance card showed a drawing of a pair of hands at prayer along with the prayer, "God grant me the Serenity to accept the things I cannot change ...Courage to change the things I can and Wisdom to know the difference."

The other side of the card stated:

God saw you getting tired, and a cure
was not to be. So he put his arms around
you, and whispered "Come to Me." With
tearful eyes we watched you, and saw
you pass away. Although we loved you
dearly, we could not make you stay. A
golden heart stopped beating, hard
working hands at rest. God broke out [sic]
hearts to prove to us, He only
takes the best.

Two Days Later

On the way to Maude's house, I stopped at the Ace Hardware store and picked up the two storm windows. I arrived at her house at 1:50. The door was unlocked, so I went in, calling out, "Maude.

Hello." I didn't hear any response and thought Maude was probably taking a nap. She wasn't in the kitchen. I went into the hallway, continuing to call out. Then I heard a reply.

"Where are you, Maude? This is Joe. I've brought the windows."

"I'm here in the living room."

I went into the living room, and she was sitting in the recliner reading.

After we exchanged pleasantries, I said, "I see you're reading something, Maude."

"I was reading my diary—what I wrote when Rusty was first starting to get sick."

"Your diary? Boy! I bet there's some good stuff in there," I smiled.

"He was always a lot of fun to be around, but then he started getting sick, and he really suffered."

"What disease did he have there at the start of his illness?"

"Alzheimer's. He began to be overly cautious while driving a car. And then he ran into that store."

"I brought the windows. I'll go ahead and bring them in and install them for you."

"All right. Go ahead. I'm getting ready to watch Doctor Laura."

"What time does she come on?"

"At two o'clock."

I went out to my car and brought in the two windows. I got Maude's Windex bottle and a roll of paper towels and washed and dried both sides of each window. As I was getting ready to install them, Maude came into the kitchen, using her walker. Within minutes I had them installed. I first raised the lower window, removed the screen, put in the upper storm window, reinstalled the screen, and positioned the lower storm window in the upper position, resting it on the flanged openings of the channels.

"There, that's it," I told her. "Everything's all set."

I sat down and took the Ace Hardware bill out of my pocket. It came to $42.68. I explained the bill to her: how I had to deposit $5, and how they deducted $5 from the final bill in order to pay me back my $5 deposit.

"Will you take a check?"

"Sure," I smiled.

"How do you spell your last name again?" she asked.

Minutes later she handed me the check.

"Thanks, Maude. You know, your one-track windows are really great, once you get the hang of them," I told her.

"Yes, I like them. I've taken down the storm windows and put them up again now for years. I've never had any trouble with them."

I was beginning to feel a bit sad that I soon would be leaving her, maybe never to see her again. I had really grown to like Maude. I thought of the first time I was at her house. I was sitting in the kitchen opposite her at the table and her son Justin came in, and I was telling him, "I fell in love with Maude the minute I saw her." I was speaking figuratively, of course, but I had really grown fond of her despite how both Rustylynn and Sarah bad-mouthed her. I never once even came close to clashing with Maude.

"Well, I'm going in to watch Doctor Laura," she said. "Then at three o'clock I go out to get the mail."

"Can I come and watch her with you?"

"Sure, if you want to."

"I'll bring the window-washing materials and maybe wash a window or two in the living room."

We went to the living room, and Maude sat down in her chair and turned on Doctor Laura. I made myself busy washing the four tiny windows in the upper part of her front door. I didn't want to start washing the other living room windows. For one thing, I didn't think Maude would want me to. When I was finished, I put away the Windex and the roll of paper towels and sat down in a straight-backed chair fairly close to Maude's chair and began to watch Doctor Laura with her. I kept thinking that I should leave, but I felt sorry for her that she had to watch the program by herself. I sat there watching it with her until the program ended at 3 o'clock.

We chatted a bit during the commercials. I told her how much I enjoyed meeting her son Richard, and her daughters, Janet and Charlotte, and Janet's son, Mark, and daughter, Hattie. She told me how Hattie is going with this guy, living with him for a while, then living by herself, and how she doesn't want to marry him, lest that might destroy their relationship.

We started walking slowly toward the kitchen, and I told her how much I liked Richard.

"Richard is autistic. People take advantage of

him."

"I enjoyed meeting the couple he lives with: Henry and Mae."

We headed into the kitchen. "I'll go out to get the mail with you," I told her. I somehow didn't want to leave. "Can you make it down the steps all right?"

"Yes, I can get down them just fine. I have another walker out in the garage."

Before leaving the kitchen, she pressed the remote to raise the garage door.

I went outside first and went into the garage and got her walker and brought it to her.

Seeing how readily I got the walker, she said, "You sure don't need a walker, do you?"

"No," I laughed.

She walked slowly with her walker to the mailbox by the curb at the intersection. "How was the funeral and lunch?" I asked.

She laughed. "We had steak for lunch, and I had a time eating it. My lower partial doesn't chew steak very good. I had to leave most of mine."

When we reached the mailbox, she opened it and withdrew the mail. "It's all junk mail," she said.

Walking slowly back toward the house I asked, "What kind of bushes are these?"

"Weigela." She pronounced it "why-jeelya."

She said the bushes flower beautifully in the spring. "Would you like a cutting?"

"A cutting?"

She broke off a sprig and gave it to me. "You

just have to dip this in some starting powder and then put it in some soil in a little pot, and then in the spring, plant it wherever you want it. I'll show you how to do it."

We went in the garage and she started down the stairway into the basement.

"I didn't know you could get into the basement this way," I said.

"Sure. I keep a key hidden right here."

"Can you get down the steps okay?"

"Yes. I do it all the time."

She went down the steps and withdrew a key from under a small box and unlocked the door. I followed her into the basement. I watched her dip the sprig into some white powder and plant it in a small pot. "There. You can take this home and give it to your wife."

"Thanks, Maude."

We headed back up the steps into the garage. She picked up a plastic container of garbage.

"Want me to put that in the garbage can for you?"

She handed me the bag and reached up above a shelf and dragged down four more bags of garbage.

"These are bags of garbage that Rustylynn put here before she left."

I put them into the garbage can.

We walked slowly out of the garage. Maude was heading for her back door to go inside.

"Well, Maude. Guess I'll be going. Now, you be sure and call me if you think I can help you do anything."

"Okay," she laughed.

"Maybe I can come over and watch Doctor Laura with you," I smiled.

"You can come over anytime you want," she said.

She opened the door to go inside, and I turned and got in my car to leave.

Eleven Days Later

"Hello, Joe?"

"Yes, this is Joe. Who's calling?" I asked.

"This is Justin, Rusty's and Maude's son."

I recognized the name right away: the son who lives nearby and who runs the business formerly owned and operated by Rusty.

"I just wanted to call and thank you for visiting my father before he died and for doing so much around the house for my mother."

"Justin, it's so nice of you to call. Let me tell you, it was a great privilege to get to know Rusty. I'm glad I was assigned to him while he was still coherent enough to conduct somewhat of a conversation. And, it was a real joy to be able to do a few things around the house to help your mother."

"Well, I can't tell you how much I appreciate what you did. Another reason I called was to ask just how I would go about making a contribution to the hospice organization. I was so very pleased with the way the hospice helped us during my father's last days."

"I know the hospice accepts contributions, but I don't know just how you go about doing this. I

298

suggest you call them. Whoever is in charge at the moment will be able to tell you how to contribute. But as to whether or not you should contribute, that's strictly up to you. If it will make you feel good inside to contribute, then by all means do so. But there's no obligation."

"Okay, I'll give them a call."

"You know, regarding my fixing things around the house for Maude, I had myself worried there for a while," I laughed. "When it was all said and done, I looked back on the whole thing and told myself: Joe, maybe you shouldn't have tackled some of those repair projects. You could have screwed something up big time!"

"Well, you didn't screw anything up. You did a magnificent job on everything you fixed."

"When I tackled that bathroom ceramic tile repair, I began to wonder if I was getting in over my head. I was a bit worried about putting in that white tile at the end of the tub when I couldn't find a replacement for the pattern of tile that was there. But I remember getting your okay before putting it in."

"Your tile repair was perfect. And that white tile looks great. It's a good match."

"And, I learned something about your single-track storm windows. Once I got the hang of them, I decided, hey, these are really neat! But I never would have figured them out if you hadn't come over that morning and got me started. I really enjoyed meeting your family at your father's wake. Especially your brother, Richard. I told Maude: 'I'll bet Richard is your favorite.'"

Justin laughed. "Janet was my father's

favorite."

"You know, that's funny. Maude told me, 'I don't have any favorites. But if I did have one, it would probably be Janet. She and I see eye to eye on everything, and we get along real good. We like each other's company.' I really like your mother. I got along good with her." I laughed. "It's kind of funny that both caregivers, Rustylynn and her sister Sarah, couldn't get along with Maude at all. Rustylynn told me, 'If it weren't for my deep faith in God, I would walk out of here and not come back. But I just turn everything over to God. I just don't let her bother me. But she is so controlling.' And, that one day I was there and Rustylynn told me, 'That woman has me right on the edge. I'm almost ready to walk out of here.' And I told her, 'Hey, why don't you get in your car and go some place and cool off. Go shopping, take a walk, or whatever. I'll stay here until you come back.' And she did. She came back three hours later refreshed and willing to get back to caring for Rusty and not let Maude bother her."

Justin laughed. "Yeah, I know. How do you like being a hospice volunteer?"

"I've been doing this for almost two years, and I really like it. Each patient situation is unique. That is, with each new patient, I sort of have to think my way through how I can best be of help. Like, with your father's situation, I quickly realized I couldn't do much for him, especially when you brought in a full-time caregiver, so I thought maybe I could be of help to Maude. When I asked her if I could do anything around the house to be of help, she said, yes, I could tighten the toilet seat. While doing that, I noticed the loose tile behind the toilet and later the broken tile around the bathtub. That led to caulking around the bathroom sink. Then came other chores for her: replacing the broken garage window; correcting the improperly installed storm windows in the kitchen and in your father's bedroom and on the south side of the southeast bedroom; reinstalling the multiple electrical outlet by the kitchen stove; fixing the leaky kitchen faucet."

"Well, I sure do appreciate everything you did."

I laughed. "Your mother just couldn't understand why I wouldn't accept any money for my labor. She told me twice, 'I've never met anyone like you before.'"

"I've been getting into some volunteer work, too. I'm doing some of that with our Lions Club. And, they're trying to get me to run for village trustee. But that would be a headache, what with all the local opposition to expanding the airport."

I told Justin I've volunteered to be on call for hospice to go to homes that request a hospice volunteer when a loved one is dying. "I'm going in for training this week."

"That's wonderful. I've been right there when ten different people have passed."

"You have? I know your first wife died, and your son, also. Were you right there when they died?"

"Yes. My wife died of cancer, and my son died of an epileptic seizure. And I was there when my father died."

We chatted for a while longer. I complimented

Justin for the mighty bur oak trees growing in his yard and also in Maude's yard. He said the trees are part of what used to be a forest of oaks in the area. "One was cut down recently, and I asked for and was given a slab of the trunk. I counted over a hundred and fifty rings in it."

Finally, Justin said, "Let me know if there's anything I can do for you."

"I spoke to your two women employees at the wake. They said they've been working for you for about fourteen years or so. I told them maybe some time they could give me a tour of your business."

"Sure, that would be fine. Come on over any time."

"And, maybe there's one more thing. Maybe you could hire me part-time working around the business. I don't know much about that kind of work, but could learn. I'm a quick learner in some things, but slow in others."

"Well, judging from your work around the house, I'd say you're a quick learner. I'll keep you in mind."

"How many people do you have working for you?"

"It varies. Anywhere from five to ten, depending on the workload."

And that was it. I told Dorothy how pleased I was that Justin had called.

Eleven Days Later

Something drew my attention to the small, white plastic pot holding the sprig of weigela

Maude had given me. It had dried up. I showed it to Dorothy.

"That looks pathetic. Why didn't you water it?"

"I did. I watered it several times. Do you suppose it's totally dead?"

"Heavens yes!"

"It doesn't have a chance of coming back to life?"

"Not a chance!"

I pulled the sprig out of the dirt and tossed it in a wastebasket. I took the pot outside and dumped the dirt in a flower bed.

Walt

Wednesday, Visit 1

The hospice office called shortly after noon to assign me a new patient: Walt, 84, advanced dementia, sleeps most of the time, and is hard of hearing. His wife, Doris, a licensed practical nurse, likes to swim. She had a caregiver but was dissatisfied and let her go. They have two sons and two daughters. The hospice office suggests I could be of help by sitting with Walt to permit Doris to get out of the house to swim or to do whatever.

I called the residence at 12:45 and spoke with Doris. I suggested I meet with her in her home at 3 o'clock this afternoon to determine how I as a volunteer could be of help. She agreed.

I pulled into the driveway at a few minutes to 3, finding the house easily. I no sooner stopped my car than a black cat appeared out of nowhere on the hood of my car, looking at me through the windshield. What the dickens! Where in the heck did that cat come from? A black one at that! Is this some kind of omen?

I got out of my car, deliberately walking around the back of the car to avoid the cat. I headed for the back door, turning to look back at my car for the cat. The cat was gone. Oh, well. As I approached the door, a voice called out, "Joe?"

"Yes, it's Joe. And, you must be Doris?"

"Yes, come on in," she said, opening the door

for me.

I stepped inside, and a black cat hopped up onto a kitchen table.

"I see you've already met my cat. You're going to have cat prints on your car," she smiled.

"Is this your cat?" I asked, referring to the cat on the table.

"Yes."

"Is this the same cat that was on my car?"

"Yes."

"I didn't see it come in. I guess it came in behind me. I'll be darned." Hey, this is some cat. It greets me on the hood of my car and then goes in the house with me without my even seeing it!

"What's its name?" I asked.

"Ghost."

"Ghost? That's a nice name for a black cat. Can I pet it?"

"Sure. It likes to be petted."

I reached out a hand and gently rubbed a finger behind its ears. It indicated approval by nudging up against my hand.

Doris was about an inch shorter than I. Her brown hair had an abundance of curls, as though she recently had a permanent. She had a matronly figure, not thin and not fat. She had a soft-spoken voice. She was wearing a gray sweatshirt and dark slacks.

"Come in and sit down," she said, leading me to a chair and table on one side of the living room. I sat at the end of the table, and Doris sat at my left. I wondered if this was a dining room table. The cat appeared quickly on top of the table, perching in front of us almost as though it were monitoring our meeting.

"Is it a female?" I don't know what made me ask this.

"Yes."

"How old is she?"

"Six years."

I reached in my pocket and brought out my hospice badge and handed it to her.

"Here's my hospice identification, just to show you I'm really a volunteer," I laughed. She took it and looked at my picture.

"I didn't know you were supposed to have a badge."

"I'm supposed to wear it, but usually just carry it in my pocket and show it as needed."

She handed the badge back to me.

"It's funny, but I've driven past your house many times but never noticed it," I said. "How long have you lived here?"

"Since 1953."

"All that time in the same house?"

"Yes."

"My goodness! What kind of work did your husband used to do?"

"He's a mechanical engineer."

"Where did he work?"

She mentioned the name of the company and its location.

"He worked there for forty-one years."

"My goodness!"

"The hospice office said you have two sons

and two daughters."

"Yes. We have a son and a daughter in nearby towns, a son in Phoenix, and a daughter in California."

"A son in Phoenix? Where does he live in Phoenix? I was raised in Phoenix."

"I can't remember the address. I'll get it."

She left me alone with the cat. I again began petting it behind its ears. It leaned into my hand. Doris returned and read the address.

"I know approximately where your son lives. It would be near what we used to call the North Mountains."

"Yes, he has a mountain real close to his house."

Somehow Doris mentioned she had been to the Casa, a Franciscan retreat house on the northeast side of Phoenix.

"The Casa?" I exclaimed. "I've been there. I went to school with the priest who used to be in charge there. This was about fifteen years ago. His name was Father Forrest."

"Father Forrest? That name isn't familiar. Did you know a Father Cecil Putakin?"

"That name is familiar. I think I've met him."

"He used to be at a church in a nearby town, but he went out to the Casa."

I suddenly recalled that I had had my first charismatic experience at the Casa.

"Are you familiar with the Charismatic Renewal?" I asked.

"Yes. I used to go to prayer meetings, but dropped out."

"Is that right. So did I. I went to the Casa one evening while I was staying at the Mountain Shadows resort nearby. A charismatic priest said mass that evening and prayed over everyone, and they all fell down. But I didn't keel over. Then after mass, a woman came up to the priest and said she wanted to be prayed over again, that she didn't feel as though she had received quite enough prayers. So the priest prayed over her again, and she keeled over again."

"Did you go to prayer meetings around here?" she asked.

"Yes, we had one at our church, and I started going to a regional prayer meeting."

"At the Haven?"

"Yes. I became one of the group's leaders. But I dropped out after having a dispute with one of the sisters. Oh, what was her name?"

"Sister Josephine?"

"Yes. You mean you know Sister Josephine?"

"Yes, I had a disagreement with her myself."

"You did? I guess a lot of people have tangled with Sister Josephine. As one of the prayer group leaders, I used to give teachings, and she didn't like one of my teachings. In my teaching, I strongly hinted that Jesus knew he was divine. Sister Josephine and another sister told me Jesus didn't know he was divine until after his resurrection."

"After his resurrection? That isn't right. Jesus said he and the Father were one."

"Yes, I know. When the sisters told me that, I decided I had to drop out of the prayer meeting, that they didn't know their theology. Tell me about your children."

"My daughter who lives in a nearby town is a psychologist."

"Is she a Ph.D?"

"Yes. She has her doctorate."

"Wow. That's really neat."

I unintentionally interrupted her.

"How long has your husband been on hospice?"

"For about a month."

"The hospice office didn't say he has a disease. He doesn't have cancer does he?"

"No. He doesn't appear to have a disease."

"Just old age, perhaps?"

"I think so."

"Does he get up and walk around?"

"No, he's bedridden. But I had him in a wheelchair earlier today and brought him in the living room."

"Is he difficult to get out of bed?"

"Not too much. He can bear some of his own weight."

"Is he eating and drinking?"

"Yes. But he tends to choke on liquids. I add a thickening agent to his liquids to ease his swallowing."

I heard a cough from across the living room, probably from a bedroom.

"Well, how can I be of help?" I asked. "The hospice office suggested perhaps I could sit with Walt to permit you to get out of the house, to swim, to shop, or to whatever.?"

"I think that would be fine, if you could stay with him for a while so I can get out."

Several more coughs came from across the living room.

"I better go see what he wants," she said, leaving me to pet Ghost again.

"Hey, Ghost, you're a real smart cat. If Dorothy weren't so allergic to cats, I'd like to take you home with me." She looked at me in such a way as to suggest, Go home with you? What makes you think I would want to do a silly thing like that? I'm happy here!

Minutes later Doris called out. "Joe, would you like to meet Walt?"

"I would love to."

I hurried across the living room and turned into a bedroom on my right. Ghost beat me in there and hopped up on a table on the right side of the room. Walt was lying on his back in a hospital bed on my left.

Doris leaned down and spoke into his left ear. "Dear, I want you to meet Joe. He's a hospice volunteer and will be staying with you every now and then."

I went up and grasped his right hand. It was ice cold.

"Hi, Walt. Nice to meet you."

Walt looked at me blankly.

"He didn't hear you," Doris said. She leaned down to speak into his left ear again. "Joe said he was glad to meet you, dear."

"I'm glad to meet him," he said gruffly.

He had white hair and a small face. I thought

that in his younger days he must have been very handsome.

"He looks as though he's really tall. Is he about six-foot-four?"

"No. He's only six feet."

"I guess if I'm going to talk to him, I have to speak into his ear."

"Yes, and speak into his left ear. He can't hear out of his right ear."

I went up to him, grasped his hand again, and bent over so my mouth was next to his left ear.

"How are you, Walt?"

"Fine."

"It's nice to meet you."

"You, too."

Then he muttered something I didn't make out. Doris came up to him.

"Did you say something is wrong with your head?" she asked him.

"No."

"What did you say, dear?"

"I want some 7-Up."

"Oh, all right."

She went to a table off to the right and brought back a glass with a straw. "He loves 7-Up."

"Well, let's see. Today's Wednesday. How about if I come over and sit with Walt tomorrow?"

"Morning or afternoon?"

"How about morning? I tend to be a morning person."

"Me too. Morning will be fine," she smiled.

"What time? About ten o'clock?"

"That would be great."

"That will allow you to go swim at the gym." The gym is an exercise/athletic facility nearby.

"Yes. I like to take part in exercise classes there, too."

"Okay, it's a deal. I'll be here tomorrow morning at ten. You can think up things for me to do for Walt while I'm here."

"You won't have much to do. He'll probably be asleep the whole time. Bring a book."

"Okay. I've got lots of reading material. Or I could feed him. Whatever."

Walt appeared to drift off to sleep, and we went back into the living room.

"The hospice office said you're a nurse. Are you an RN?"

"No. I'm an LPN, a licensed practical nurse."

She proceeded to spell out the differences between an RN and an LPN.

"I used to work at a nuns' mother house."

"Taking care of retired sisters?"

"Yes."

"Sisters can really live to a ripe old age, can't they?"

"Boy, they sure can! That's because they never married," she laughed.

"Then I guess you've been around a lot of dying patients?"

"Yes, lots of them."

I told her about my recent experience with a hospice patient where a caregiver was giving the patient permission to "go and be with his mother."

"I've done that with some of the dying sisters—given them permission to die. It makes it a lot easier for them to die."

"Barbara told me you had a full-time caregiver for a while but it didn't work out."

"Yes. It was a woman from a European country. She couldn't speak a word of English. We just could not communicate with each other. I'm going to try being without a caregiver for a while."

Minutes later I was heading for my car. I looked around for Ghost. I thought sure she came out the door with me. Where had she gone? I got in my car and looked at my hood. No Ghost. I looked around inside the car. No Ghost. Oh, well. I headed home.

What a joy to meet Doris and Walt. I was looking forward to tomorrow to sit with Walt. My goodness, it's only been two days since I attended the funeral of my last hospice patient!

Driving home I thought about Walt. He doesn't look good. He isn't swallowing very good. His hands are icy.

Thursday, Visit 2

At 9:50 I parked on the right side of the driveway in front of the two-car garage. I wondered if maybe I should have parked on the left side. Which side of the garage does she have her car parked? But then, wait a minute. Didn't Doris say she was going to the gym to swim? She most likely would walk.

Getting out of the car, I saw her plastic recycle bin upside down near the curb. I decided to bring it in for her. As I bent over to pick it up, I must have bumped the alarm button on my car's keyless entry security module in my pocket, because the horn alarm on my car became activated. Beep! Beep! Beep! ...Embarrassed, I whipped out the module and pressed the alarm button, deactivating it. The horn stopped!

I carried the recycle bin to the back porch and set it down, and Doris came to the door.

"That darn car alarm. I just bent over to pick up your recycle bin and somehow activated it! Oh, brother!"

"They're handy to have when you can't find your car in a parking lot," she laughed.

"Are you going swimming?"

"No, I have a lot of errands to do."

"Oh, okay. So you'll be using your car. I parked on the right side of the driveway. Is that all right?"

"Yes, because my car is on the left side of the garage. My son's car is on the right side."

"Let me go out and move my car a bit farther to the right to make it easy for you to back out."

I hurried outside and moved my car a bit to the right.

"Where's Ghost?" I asked, back inside the house.

"Oh, she's somewhere in the house asleep. Probably down in the basement."

I followed her into Walt's bedroom to receive instructions. Walt was lying on his back and was sleeping soundly. His mouth was wide open, and his withdrawn cheeks made his face look very old. His white hair was thinning at the forehead. His sheets were pale green, and he was covered to his chest with an off-white blanket. He was wearing a green, blue, and white plaid buttoned shirt with long sleeves.

"He probably will sleep the whole time I'm gone. But if he wakes up, you can offer him some 7-Up. If he says he's hungry, there's some Jell-O in the refrigerator. There's the remote for his bed, so you can raise the head of his bed. He's had his breakfast, and I've got him all cleaned up."

Heading back toward the kitchen, Doris said, "He's been talking to his mother this morning."

"Is that right? Does he usually do that?"

"No."

"Another caregiver told me that shortly before the end, her patients almost always start communicating with spirits, usually family members."

"I might be gone for some time," she said apologetically.

"That's all right. Take as long as you want. I don't have to be anywhere."

"Oh, here's a flyer I received recently in the mail from the Casa," she said. Then she said good-bye and went out the back door and headed for the garage.

I went to the dining room table and sat down and started to read my book, "Filth Eater," by Stanley L. Struble, alumni director at Boys Town. He self-published it and sent me an autographed copy a few days ago with a note that said it had yet to be proofread. I took it on myself to proofread it for him. Stanley and I are both graduates of Boys Town: he in 1968, and myself in 1947. We began corresponding a year ago when he mailed back one of my manuscripts I had submitted to Boys Town for review. He subsequently had me proofread three of his manuscripts, including "Filth Eater." He really writes well. His stories, replete with adventure and intrigue, concern archeologists in the Mayan-Aztec regions of Mexico and Guatemala.

The table, flush against the north wall of the living room, is covered with a green tablecloth. Vertical blinds are on the window by the table. Above the table is a small chandelier with eight candle lights and hanging tear drop crystals.

I glanced around the living room and admired the bookcase-like partition isolating the front door. Vertical blinds are also on the big bay window on the west side of the living room. The south side of the living room has a sofa, two end tables with lamps and a big wall painting of a seashore. The east wall of the living room has a fire place, TV, an armrest chair, and a statue of St. Francis (or St. Anthony?).

After reading a dozen or so pages, I heard Walt cough several times. I went in to look at him. He was still sleeping soundly, so I went back to my reading. After additional coughs, I made several more trips to check on him. Finally I closed my book and decided to go into the bedroom and spend some time with him.

He was beginning to cough frequently. It was as though he was aspirating slightly. The coughing was an apparent attempt to clear his throat. I began to notice that his breathing was raspy and gurgly. He was beginning to moan between his coughs. Maybe if I would raise the head of his bed, this would allow the throat fluids to go down and ease his breathing.

I picked up the remote. Should I raise the head of his bed and awaken him? Walt must have read my mind, because he opened his eyes slightly.

"Hi, Walt. Did you wake up? I'm going to raise the head of your bed. I think you would like that. It ought to make it easier for you to breathe."

As I raised his head, he began to stare at me through half-raised eyelids. Raising his head did seem to reduce his coughing, probably by helping drain fluids from his throat.

"Henrietta!" he called out.

"Henrietta? Who's that?" I asked him. "My name is Joe, and I'm here to take care of you while Doris goes shopping," I said. Then I remembered that he's hard of hearing and it is necessary to speak into his left ear. I moved the portable tray away from his bed and went up to him and bent over to speak into his ear, repeating what I had just said.

He didn't say anything but continued to look at me suspiciously. I bent down by his ear and repeated what I had said. Still no response.

"Henrietta!" he called out again.

"Who is Henrietta?" I asked him, speaking into his ear.

No response.

"Would you like some 7-Up, Walt?"

"Yes," he blurted.

I reached for the 7-Up on his tray and offered it to him, placing the tip of the straw into his mouth. He started to suck on the straw and brought up both hands to hold the can. Doris had the can inside of a plastic cup, which she had told me helps keep the 7-Up cold. After a few sips, he moved the can away from him, signaling for me to take it.

"Was that good, Walt? Do you like 7-Up?"

No response. He probably hadn't heard me, as I hadn't spoken into his left ear. His eyelids drooped shut as though he were going back to sleep.

I looked down at his urine bag. It had been turned around so the white plastic side of the bag was facing me. I bent down and looked behind the bag to see his urine. It was dark.

When I stood up Walt was looking at me again. The poor thing, he probably wonders who I am. I reached down and grasped his right hand with my right hand, and his left hand with my left hand. I tugged gently on each hand, as though I were trying to pull him forward. He seemed to like what I was doing. I did this several times and then let go of his hands. Maybe he would like for me to put my arm around his back and sit him up straight. I thought about this for a few seconds and decided not to. I didn't want to do anything like that without first checking with Doris.

"Henrietta!" he called out once again.

"Who is Henrietta?"

No response.

With Walt still looking at me, I went around to the foot of his bed and began gently massaging his feet through his black socks.

"Does that feel good, Walt?"

No response. He doesn't hear me. He kept staring at me. I decided to offer him some more 7-Up. I picked up the can and brought it to him. He saw it coming and reached out to hold it. I put the straw into his mouth. The can felt as though it was about empty. When he gave the can back to me, I took the can out of the mug and shook it. It was practically empty!

I went to the kitchen and opened the refrigerator and found an unopened can of 7-Up. There was Ghost sitting near the back door. I called her, but got no response. I took the 7-Up into the bedroom.

"I've got you a new can of 7-Up, Walt. Wait till I pop the lid, and stick the can in the mug, then you can have some."

I transferred the straw from the empty can to the full one. As I was about to place the mug in his hands, I inadvertently nudged the tip of the straw, and it swung around, hurling a drop of 7-Up into the corner of his left eye.

"You've got 7-Up in my eye," he rebelled loudly, grimacing as though in pain and rubbing his eye with his fingers.

I reached for a tissue from a box on a nearby table and wiped at his eye. I bent down to speak into his ear.

"There, Walt. I'm sorry."

"That's okay," he replied.

Hey, now we're communicating! He took a few

sips and I put the can back on the tray. I bent down to his ear again.

"How old are you, Walt?"

"Eighty-four," he said without hesitation.

"And, when is your birthday?"

The date he told me was correct.

Hadn't Barbara told me he had Alzheimer's? How could that be? This man is quite rational!

"What's your middle name, Walt?"

"Antonio."

"Antonio? Are you Italian?"

"Yes. I'm Italian."

"Are you Catholic?"

"Yes."

I stood up straight and looked down at his face. His eyelids drooped about a fourth shut. How smooth his facial skin looked. I guess Doris probably shaves him every day. I tried to think up more questions to ask him. I bent down to his ear again.

"My name is Joe. I'm here to stay with you while your wife goes shopping."

"Hi, Joe."

"I'm Joe-Joe from Kokomo, riding on a buffalo." I thought this might trigger a smile. It got no response. I repeated it a couple of times. No response.

I felt the urge to sneeze and sneezed into my handkerchief.

"God bless you," he said.

"Thanks, Walt." I sneezed again, but this time I got silence.

He periodically raised his knees and strained, as though he were experiencing gastro-intestinal cramps. After one such episode, I bent down to his ear.

"Are you in pain, Walt?"

No response.

I wondered what his pulse was. I put my fingers on the inside of his wrist and felt for a pulse. I couldn't seem to detect one. Maybe if I would put my fingers along his carotid artery on his neck. I looked at his neck. It was thin, with bulging cords. I looked at his eyes. I bent over to his ear.

"Do you have brown eyes, Walt?"

No response.

"How tall are you, Walt?"

"Five foot one." I'm sure he meant *six* foot one.

"How much do you weigh?"

"One hundred seventy-two."

Now we're really communicating again.

"Are you an engineer?"

No response. I began to study the big picture on the wall behind the head of his bed. It was titled, "Garden Birds," and had paintings of a couple dozen birds one is likely to see in a yard. Beautiful. It made me wish I had got into birding.

I glanced around the room. A computer was in the southwest corner. I wondered if Walt used to operate it. A large picture of Jesus was on the west wall. It was a modern portrait, with Jesus smiling broadly, his hair tussled, making him look very macho, as though he were "one of the guys." Somehow I didn't care for it. The painting was well done, but I just couldn't picture Jesus that way. I'm too used to seeing him in a serious pose.

I offered him more 7-Up, and he took a few sips. I was extra careful not to whip the top of the straw around so as to avoid getting another drop in his eye.

I wondered if he was cold. I checked the temperature setting on the wall thermostat in the hallway right outside his bedroom door. It was set on 69. I felt Walt's hands. They felt nice and warm. What a contrast to when I was here yesterday when his hands were icy. While grasping his hands, I again tugged gently, as though trying to sit him up. He seemed to find this a pleasant preoccupation.

I heard the back door open. Doris had returned. I looked at my watch. It was 11:55. She had been gone for two hours. Two hours? Where had the time gone? It seemed as though she had just left. I went into the kitchen, where Doris was placing a few grocery bags on the sink counter.

"You're back! Did you get all your errands done?"

"Yes. Thanks so much, Joe. I sure appreciate it. How was he?"

We headed for the bedroom.

"He was just fine. He started coughing and rasping, so I raised the head of his bed. I gave him the rest of the 7-Up in the can by his bed and got him a new can out of the refrigerator. I was having fun talking with him. We were communicating pretty good. I don't think he has Alzheimer's."

"No, he doesn't have Alzheimer's."

"The hospice office said he might have a touch of it. But I don't think he does. He's quite rational."

Doris bent down to speak into his ear.

"Did Joe take good care of you?"

I stood at the foot of his bed looking at him.

"Who is this guy?" Walt blurted out.

"This is Joe. He's here to take care of you."

I laughed. "Who is this guy? That's funny. Who is this guy? I told him who I was, but I guess he didn't understand. Maybe I didn't say it loud enough."

"He seems to be shivering. He must be cold," Doris said. She reached for a blanket and spread it over him.

"I felt his hands several times, and they always felt quite warm. Could he perhaps be frightened of me?" I smiled.

"That could be."

We went into the living room, and Doris showed me several books she bought at Crown Books. I showed her "Filth Eater," the inscription inside the front page from the author. I explained what it was about.

"When would you like for me to come back and sit with Walt again?"

"I might need you again next week."

"Okay. I'm pretty well freed up except on Tuesday, when I sit with my Alzheimer's patient. Please don't hesitate to use me. Seriously, I want you to call on me anytime."

"Okay. Give me your phone number."

I wrote my name and phone number on a piece of paper and gave it to her.

"Is he in diapers?" I asked.

"I put him in diapers sometimes, but right now I don't have any on him. He has the catheter in, and I have protective pads under him. It's easy to clean him up without the diapers on him."

"He called out several times for Henrietta. You had mentioned that he was calling for his mother. Is Henrietta his mother?"

"No," she smiled. "Henrietta is his sister. She's a year older than he is, and she lives with my daughter."

"I sneezed and Walt said, 'God bless you.' I thought that was pretty neat."

Doris laughed.

When I got home I told Dorothy about Walt asking his wife, "Who is this guy?" She laughed.

That night in bed I thought about my visit with Walt. It was a bit tough to begin communicating with him, but we got along well. I laughed again at his asking his wife, "Who is this guy?"

Saturday, Visit 3

Doris phoned at 11:45 and asked if I could come over as soon as practicable and sit with Walt while she went to a travel agency to pick up a plane ticket for her daughter. I told her, sure, I would be right over. I quickly finished eating my lunch, poured my hot tea into my Thermos, and set out for the house.

I arrived at 12:10, parking well to the right side of the driveway so she could back her car out. Carrying my Thermos and looking around and not seeing Ghost, I went to the back door, and Doris let me in. I slipped off my jacket and draped it around the back of a chair at the table with the green tablecloth in the living room just outside the kitchen.

"He's much worse now than he was when you last saw him," she said. "He's asleep and shouldn't wake up. Don't go into his room, it might disturb him."

"Okay. You don't want me to go into his room? Is there anything you want me to do while you're gone?"

"Just be here," she smiled.

I sat down at the opposite side of the table from where I had draped my jacket over a chair. Doris picked up my jacket, thinking it was hers.

"Oh, no. This is your jacket."

"That's okay. You can wear it if you want," I laughed.

She went into her bedroom and returned with her coat and put it on. She picked up her purse from the table when Walt coughed.

"Oh-oh. He's waking up," she said, stopping in her tracks. "I better give him some medicine." She took off her coat and laid it on the table and went into Walt's bedroom.

I sat at the table and poured my tea into my Thermos cup and began to drink it. I sat there for a few minutes and decided to go to Walt's bedroom and look in. Doris was on Walt's left giving him some medicine.

"Can I come in?"

"Sure," she replied.

I went into the bedroom and stood on Walt's right. He turned to look at me. His eyelids were drooped half shut.

"He doesn't look so good. I took his teeth out so he can breathe better."

Without his teeth, his mouth puckered inward. He was wearing another plaid shirt. I could see a T-shirt underneath. A blanket covered him to his chest. His right hand was under the blanket.

"Hi, Walt," I said, speaking softly. I knew he didn't hear me, but he was looking straight at me. Doris bent down to speak into his left ear.

"This is Joe. He's a nurse. He's going to stay with you while I go to the store."

I'm a nurse? That's a new one. Walt mumbled something but it was so faint it was impossible to make out what he was saying.

"Can I stay in here with him while you're gone? I'll just hold his hand and talk to him very softly."

Doris looked at Walt for a few moments.

"I guess it will be all right. My daughter stayed here last night and we were holding his hand much of the night. He had a temperature last night. I think he was coming down with something when you were here before."

Doris came around to the side of the bed where I was and picked up the straw from the 7-Up can on the bed tray. She placed the wet end of the straw into Walt's mouth, then put the straw back into the can.

"Do you think it would help if you raised the head of his bed? Would that make it easier for him to breathe?" I asked.

"Okay."

Doris picked up the remote and raised the head of his bed a little ways.

"I'll be back as soon as I can," she said and left the bedroom to make her way out of the house to her car in the garage.

"I'll be right back, Walt. I want to get my cup of tea." I had left it on the table with the green tablecloth.

I set my cup on the tray on the right side of Walt's bed and pulled back the blanket to find his right hand. I remembered that Doris had told me she usually left Walt without a diaper on. I grasped his hand with my right hand and restored the blanket to where it was.

"Walt, let me raise the head of your bed a bit for you."

I picked up the remote and raised his head all the way. He looked uncomfortable, so I backed it down slightly.

"There, Walt, now you look comfortable. I'll leave it right there."

I grasped his right hand again with my right hand, and with my left hand, picked up my cup and finished my tea.

"Okay, Walt, what can we talk about?"

Walt began to mumble something faintly. I had no idea what he was saying. He was so weak it wasn't really even mumbling—just a barely audible noise with his lips moving ever so slightly.

I knew he couldn't hear me. But I didn't want to go around the bed and speak into his ear.

"Have you seen Henrietta?"

No response.

"Have you seen your mother?"

No response.

"Do you want to go to your mother?"

No response.

He again made the barely audible noise with his lips moving slightly.

"Are you going on a trip, Walt?"

No response.

"Are you going on vacation? To California? To Colorado? To go hunting? To hunt bear? To hunt deer? Are you going fishing? In one of those crystal-clear mountain streams with tall pines on either side?"

No response.

"Are you going to take a train? A plane?"

All the while he was looking at me.

His breathing was interrupted by a few coughs. They were terrible-sounding coughs, as though he was struggling to clear his throat. Then he resumed normal breathing.

I released his hand for a few seconds. He raised his hand up, apparently wanting me to continue holding it. I grasped his hand again and began stroking his head very softly with my left hand.

"Does that feel good, Walt?"

He continued to stare at me. I thought about

his pulse. Still holding his right hand with my right hand, I placed the fingers of my left hand on the inside of his wrist to probe for a pulse. There it was! I could feel it. It was beating rapidly. But, there, it skipped a beat. Then another, and another. About every four or five beats it would skip. Remembering to wear my watch, I looked at it to take a pulse reading. I was going to count the beats for 15 seconds and multiply by four. The skipped beats kept throwing me off. How do you take a pulse when it skips beats? Do you just count the beats? Or do you count the beats and add a beat for every skipped beat? I figured his pulse was somewhere around 100. That has to be real fast for a man of 84.

I kept holding his hand while I recited an Our Father, Hail Mary, and Glory Be. I repeated the three prayers. He kept looking at me. His eyelids were still drooped half shut. Or were they half open?

I looked out the windows at the passing cars. I watched the cars stop at a four-way stop. I wondered if the intersection ought to have a traffic signal. There was a lot of traffic entering and leaving a parking lot. I saw a woman get out of her car wearing a green workout suit and carrying a handbag.

I let go of Walt's hand again. He raised it, apparently wanting me to continue holding it. I grasped his hand again and resumed stroking his head with my left hand.

"You really want me to hold your hand, don't you, Walt?"

I felt his pulse again. Now it was beating very slowly. I counted it for 10 seconds and multiplied by six. Thirty? I felt the pulse again. Now it was beating fast again, with a lot of skipped beats. I monitored his breathing. It wasn't good. Probably twice as rapid as normal.

"Your forehead doesn't feel hot like you have a temperature, Walt." I recalled Doris saying he had had a temperature last night.

Ghost came into the room and sprang up onto the dresser a little ways from the foot of Walt's bed.

"Hi, Ghost."

She looked at me and began licking herself. Minutes later she leaped to the floor and came up to me. I let go of Walt's hand and reached down and gently rubbed behind her ears. Then she turned and left the room. I stood up and Walt was raising his hand again. I grasped it and resumed stroking his head. I was tempted to go around to the other side of the bed and speak into his good ear. But what good would that do? He can't talk anymore anyway, just make a faintly audible noise. I stayed where I was. I resumed questioning him about his "upcoming vacation trip."

I studied his nicely proportioned small features. How old he looked without his teeth! But I could tell he had been handsome in his day.

Staring at his eyes, it suddenly occurred to me his eyelids were no longer drooping. His eyes were wide open! What was this?

"Your eyes are wide open, Walt. What happened?"

I had no idea. I thought about offering him some 7-Up, or at least putting the wet end of the straw in his mouth. I better not. Doris didn't tell me to give him any 7-Up.

I looked once again at the picture of Jesus on the west wall of his bedroom. Such a macho Jesus! His dark hair was tussled. He had a stubble of dark whisker growth around his mouth and chin. He was smiling, and his eyes were dancing with life. Instead of Jesus, he looked like something out of Hollywood.

As I continued to hold Walt's hand, look into his eyes, and ponder the great meaning of life, a noise coming from the kitchen told me Doris had returned.

"Doris is back," I smiled at Walt.

I let go of his hand and went into the kitchen to greet Doris.

"How did things go?" she asked, heading for the bedroom.

"Just great," I said, following her. Doris went to the left side of Walt's bed, the side with his good ear, and I went to his right.

"I raised the head of his bed a bit, and he coughed only a couple of times. I stayed right by his side practically the whole time, holding his hand and stroking his head. I managed to find his pulse, and it's been erratic—missing a lot of beats. I can't believe how wide open his eyes are."

"I haven't seen his eyes open this wide for some time," she smiled.

"I think he likes me now. He spoke to me several times, but it was so faint I couldn't tell what he was saying."

"I can't understand him either," she said. "I think he's still running a temperature."

"His forehead feels normal to me," I said. I put my hand on his forehead again just to make sure. "Yeah, it still feels normal. I think his temperature it gone."

I let go of his hand and started to follow Doris out of the room.

"Wait, I want to say good-bye to Walt," I told her, going around to the other side of his bed. I bent down to his left ear.

"Good-bye, Walt. I have to be going now. Good-bye." I knew I was really saying good-bye forever.

I picked up my jacket from the chair by the table with the green tablecloth and told Doris, "It kind of amused me when you told Walt I was his nurse," I laughed.

"I just wanted to reassure him you were going to take good care of him."

I picked up my Thermos and noticed it was lacking its cup.

"I have to go back in the bedroom and get my cup."

Walt was still in the same position looking toward the door.

"Good-bye, Walt," I said again. But I knew he couldn't hear me.

"Thanks, Joe, for coming," Doris said.

"Did you get the plane ticket for your daughter in California?"

"Yes."

"Please don't hesitate to call me again if I can be of any help whatsoever," I reassured her.

I looked around for Ghost as I went out the

back door, but I didn't see her.

Monday

At 11:55 a.m. the hospice office called to tell me Walt died this morning. I had figured that he would die within a day or two. She said she was on her way to visit a new hospice patient and would likely be calling me back to assign him to me.

She said she has turned in her two-week notice and that Friday will be her last day. She said she has been in conflict with her management and doesn't need the stress. She likely will seek employment with another hospice. She doesn't know who will take her place.

I thanked her for her kindness to me and complimented her for her great sense of understanding in dealing with hospice volunteers.

Wednesday

Walt's obituary in this morning's newspaper gave me his funeral arrangements. I arrived at the funeral home at about 3:15. It was about 20 degrees, with a strong breeze and light snow. I signed in and picked up a remembrance card showing a painting of Jesus with a halo and with his heart surrounded by thorns with a flame coming out the top and with rays of light emanating in all directions. Jesus is wearing a white top with a red cape draped just below his shoulders and over each hand. At the bottom of the picture it states, "Sacred Heart of Jesus, Have Mercy on Us." The background is blue sky with small clouds. A fine gold line frames the picture. The back of the card states:

> I am the resurrection
> and the life, he who be-
> lieves in Me, even if he
> die, shall live; and who-
> ever lives and believes in
> Me shall not die forever.

Doris was sitting on a sofa with two ladies. I went up to her and she stood up and we chatted for a few minutes. She apologized for not calling me and said Walt died at about 7:30 Monday morning. I told her the hospice office called to tell me Walt had died. She introduced me to her daughter from California, who said she arrived Sunday.

Doris walked with me up to the casket. Walt's face looked very white. He was wearing a white shirt, dark tie, and pinstripe suit.

"Is that a navy blue suit and tie?" I asked Doris.

"I don't know if it's navy blue or black."

He had a gold pin in his lapel and a brown rosary entwined around his folded hands. The brown casket was bedecked with a beautiful array of red roses.

I knelt to say a prayer for Walt. It was nice knowing you, Walt. May God grant you a favorable spot in heaven. Thanks for letting me hold your hand Saturday.

Doris said several sisters from the mother house where she used to work were at the wake earlier. She introduced me to Walt's sister,

Henrietta, whom Walt was calling that day I was with him while Doris was going on errands. She was sitting in a wheelchair and had a pleasant smile and was very cognitive. She seemed pleased when I told her Walt had called out for her when I was sitting with him.

A few feet away was a beautiful picture of Walt and Henrietta when they were about four or five years old.

Doris then introduced me to her daughter who lives in a nearby town. I asked where Nicholas was, her son who lives in Phoenix. She said he was in the lounge having coffee and cookies.

"I want to meet him so I can talk with him about Phoenix," I told Doris.

Doris led me into the lounge, telling me that Nicholas was deaf.

"You mean I will have to speak loud for him to understand?"

"No, it's more than that. He just can't hear."

Doris spoke right into Nicholas's face, telling him I was Joe, a hospice volunteer. He nodded that he understood and muttered something. His voice did not sound clear at all. I shook his hand and caught myself staring at his pony tail.

"You don't think there's any use of my trying to chat with him about Phoenix?" I asked Doris.

"No. He won't be able to hear you."

I turned and nodded to Nicholas, and he nodded back, and I left with Doris, heading back into the parlor. I felt defeated. I had been looking forward to chatting with him about Phoenix.

"Because of Nicholas's deafness, I'm going to have a 'signer' at the funeral," Doris said.

"You mean one of those people who stand up front and move their hands for signs for the deaf?"

"Yes."

"I've met all your children except your other son," I told her.

She led me to a man sitting in a chair a few feet away.

"I understand you were with your dad when he died," I said.

"Yes."

"That's beautiful. Were you holding his hand?"

"No, I wasn't holding his hand. I was sitting in a chair by the bed. It was about seven fifteen. I had noticed that he was breathing very softly. I leaned back in the chair and closed my eyes. When I opened my eyes at about seven-thirty, he had stopped breathing."

He had long fingers like his father.

"Did Walt play the piano?" I asked.

"He used to play the piano a long time ago," Doris said.

"Our choir director always used to say men with long fingers make good piano players, and I had noticed Walt had long fingers. Mine are short," I held up my hands, "so I wouldn't make a good piano player," I laughed.

I shook hands with Doris again, telling her I would see her at the funeral. I told her I knew the pastor of the church where the funeral was to be held.

"He was just here," she said.

"Good-bye," I said, turning to leave.

Thursday

I pulled into the parking lot of the church at 9:45. It was 20 degrees, and about an inch of snow had fallen. A man who looked old enough to be retired was standing by the entry of the lot. I assumed correctly that because of the funeral he was directing traffic into the lot. He pointed to where he wanted me to park. I put down my window to ask him if I would be trapped by the funeral procession, and he said no. I recall at another funeral at this church how I was trapped in my car until the funeral procession pulled out of the lot.

I went into church and looked around in the vestibule for a snow shovel to clear off the walk in front of church. I didn't see any. I went inside the sanctuary and selected a pew half way down the left side, just as I had done at the other funeral. I took a seat near the left end of the pew.

I looked around, studying the church design. What appeared to be a large metal sculpture of Jesus holding a staff adorned the wall behind the altar. Seven beams on each side supported the steeply slanted roof. I counted 22 pews on each side of the central aisle. With a capacity of about 32 per pew row, that gave the church a seating capacity of 642. Five ceiling fans whirled high overhead. Six horizontal stained-glass windows adorned each side of the church. I wondered about the significance, if any, of 12 stained-glass windows. One for each Apostle? The 12 tribes of

Israel?

Glancing toward the altar I saw the pastor moving about getting everything ready. A few ladies were scurrying about on the right side of the altar. I presumed (correctly) they were preparing to provide the music and singing for the funeral. I wondered if I should go up and ask them if I could join them. Something told me deep inside not to do this, so I stayed in the pew.

A woman was positioning a floor microphone to the left of the lectern, and the pastor pointed to a spot where she should put it. I wondered if she was going to be a soloist. If so, why would she be across the altar from the piano.

I wondered if the hearse would arrive at the church on time. At my church, the hearse invariably gets there five to 10 minutes late. This one was early. By 9:55 the casket was in position in the back of the sanctuary, along with family members, waiting for the pastor to come to them and begin the ceremonies. Getting to the church five minutes early, and on a snowy day! Wow! This funeral home is punctual!

At 10 o'clock sharp, the pastor, wearing white vestments, and the woman who had been positioning the floor microphone came down the aisle and went to the casket. When the priest started the preliminary prayers, the woman stood by his side making hand signs for the deaf. So, she was to be the 'signer'! Only a handful of people were in the congregation. We stood and turned around to watch and listen to the proceedings. Minutes later the priest turned and led the pallbearers, casket, family members, and friends toward the altar. I recognized only one of the pallbearers: Doris's son who lives in a nearby town. I was fascinated that one of the pallbearers was a black man, and that a black lady was among the family and friends following the casket. Doris and her son from Phoenix led the small entourage following the casket. I recognized her two daughters in the group.

When the casket was halted in front of the altar, Doris followed her son Nicholas into the first pew on the left, followed by her two daughters and apparently friends, including the black man and black lady. I kept wondering who the black couple was.

The opening hymn was "Be Not Afraid," and was sung by three ladies standing off to the right of the altar accompanied by a woman at a piano. Each sang into a microphone, and their voices carried well throughout the church. I suddenly wished I was up there singing with them. The woman "signer" went through her hand motions for the words to the hymn and subsequently signed every word uttered by the pastor, the guest reader, and eulogists.

Doris's other son gave the first reading. I thought he said the reading was from Galatians 3:6-14. The singers then sang "Shepherd Me, O God" as the psalm. Since there was to be no second reading, the singers went right into the "Alleluia," for the gospel, which the celebrant said was from John. In it, Jesus tells his disciples how he has prepared places for them in heaven.

Following are excerpts from the homily: "A well-known church in Rome has a baptistry, a building as big as this church, which has doors that are so beautiful that Michelangelo said they could serve as the doors to heaven ...this goes to show the importance of baptism in the early church ...Walt rose to a new life through baptism ...making his pilgrimage through life ...Jesus is the way, the truth, and the life ...the first reading reminds us that we get to heaven by actions as well as words ...Walt lived a life of faith ...we are thanking God for the new life Walt has been called to ...he was faithful to his wife and children ...may the souls of Walt and the souls of all the faithful departed rest in peace."

The Offertory hymn was "Make Me a Channel of Your Peace."

The celebrant brought communion to each person in the left front pew. After I went forward and received communion, I kept my eyes in front of me as I walked past Doris in the front pew.

The communion hymn was "Hear I Am Lord." While the pastor swung the censor walking around the casket, the three ladies sang "Jesus, Remember Me." I recalled from my days in the choir when this priest was our pastor that this was one of his favorite songs. I guess it still is. The song repeats over and over the line, "Jesus, remember me, when you come into your kingdom."

At the conclusion of the regular services, the celebrant invited eulogists to come forward and speak. Doris's son who lives nearby went up to the microphone and spoke of his father in words that included: "My Dad was a kind, sensitive, and caring person ...he made people feel welcome in his home ...he always welcomed me with 'come in, please sit down, would you like something to drink?' ...I thank God I had such a dad, and I thank God he is at peace."

Then his wife stood up and turned around to face the congregation and spoke softly and haltingly, telling how she loved the deceased and what a fine man he was. Why didn't she go up to the microphone? I couldn't understand much of what she said.

The closing hymn was "On Eagles' Wings," sung while the family and congregation followed the casket down the aisle toward the rear of the church.

As I waited in the main aisle for the family to leave the church, the celebrant, returning to the altar, stopped to shake my hand.

"Hi, Father," I smiled, grasping his hand.

"Hi, Joe. Did you know Walt?" he asked.

"I met him as a hospice volunteer. I liked your singers. They did a really nice job."

"Thanks," he said, heading for the altar.

As I headed for my car, the funeral procession had not left. The man who had directed my parking had selected a spot for me wisely: I exited the lot without having to wait for the procession.

Nine Days Later

I received a thank-you card today, as follows:

Dear Joe,
We shall always remember
with deep gratitude
your comforting expression of sympathy.

Walt's Family

Diane

"I want to go to the eight-thirty mass on Monday. It's our sixty-third wedding anniversary," Edward says, looking up from his bent-over stance, clinging to his walker for support. "Can you take me?" He speaks softly, with a trace of a European accent.

"Your sixty-third wedding anniversary? You want to go to the eight-thirty mass on Monday? Sure, I can take you," I smile.

"I won't have any errands to run or any doctor appointments next week," he says. His blue eyes twinkle behind his rimmed glasses.

"Okay, Edward. I'll pick you up at eight-fifteen, Monday. Will that be okay?"

"Yes," he beams with appreciation.

What a joy it will be to drive this delightful gentleman to mass for his 63rd anniversary, I tell myself as I drive the six blocks to my home after taking him to the Saturday 5 o'clock mass. Edward is 89, and his wife, Diane, is 86. I am a hospice volunteer and was assigned to Diane almost five months ago shortly after she experienced difficulty in swallowing, and her doctor, declaring her terminal, recommended placing her in home hospice care. Since then her swallowing has not deteriorated further, but her overall waning physical condition along with Alzheimer's confines her to bed.

As a hospice volunteer, I normally visit and chat with my assigned patient. But in Diane's case, she has a live-in caregiver, so the best way I can be of help is to assist Edward, her spouse. In addition to driving him to weekly mass, I take him to the doctor, dentist, optometrist, audiologist, barbershop, bank, or wherever.

I also assist Edward with his memoirs, which he is writing for his children and grandchildren. Being a retired writer/editor, this is a natural for me. His life story is engaging. He and his wife emigrated from Belgium on August 27, 1938, on the very day they were married! They didn't leave any too soon, because shortly after that, Hitler's Panzer divisions swept into Belgium, the Netherlands, Luxembourg, and France.

At 8:13 Monday morning, August 27, I pull up in front of Edward's yellow brick, two-story house. A few puffy white clouds surf a blue sky toward the southwest. Commercial jets skim across the Maplewood sky in a glide path for the airport. I normally back into his driveway to make it easy for him to get into my car, but I park in the street because a car blocks the driveway. A woman stands at the front door ringing the bell. I theorize that it's the hospice nurse's aide, come to bathe Diane. I park facing south to give Edward access to my passenger door, certain that the village won't object to my parking for only a few minutes on the wrong side of the street.

The door opens to admit the nurse's aide, and Marina, the live-in caregiver, waves to me. "Hi, Marina," I wave back.

I go inside and up the three steps to the living room.

"Hi, Edward," I say. He's bent over pushing his walker in the dining room.

"Hi, Joe. I have to go to the bathroom first."

Most of the time I go to the room at the back of the house to say a few words to Diane in her hospital bed. But this morning, with the nurse's aide there to bathe her, it would not be appropriate. I sit down on the living room sofa, glancing around the room at family pictures and gazing admiringly at a tall, brown, hand-carved wooden monk. Every time I look at the monk, which Edward said his son, Charles, bought for him in Mexico, I tell myself that my wife, Dorothy, would kill for it.

About five minutes later Edward, pushing his walker, turns the corner from the bathroom to the living room.

"Are you ready to go?" I ask.

"Yes." He stops suddenly and turns to look longingly back toward Diane. Then he starts toward me. I wait until he halts his walker and grasps a brown, wooden cane leaning against a waist-high console.

"I want to put on a coat. I got cold in church Saturday," he says.

I precede him down the three steps to the small vestibule.

"Do you want me to get you a coat?" I point to the vestibule closet.

"Yes."

I open the door. A dozen or so coats, jackets, and sweaters cling limply to hangers.

"Which coat would you like?"

"That one. The blue one."

"This one?"

"Yes."

I remove the dark blue coat, sort of a combination jacket and sweater, and hand it to him.

"Can I help you with it?" I ask.

"No. I can manage."

I pick up the folded aluminum walker that he keeps by the door and carry it out to the porch and down the steps. I spread open the walker at the end of the black iron railing. I stand there and watch him, using his cane, struggle bent over out the front door and down the steps. When he reaches the walker he hands me his cane.

"I had to park on the street because the nurse's aide's car is blocking the driveway. Can you walk all the way to the street?"

"Yes."

Carrying his cane, I walk slowly ahead of him to the car. I turn and watch him maneuver the walker down the single step where his sidewalk joins the street sidewalk. I open the passenger door and, using my remote key, pop open the trunk. After he gets in, I close the door, fold up the walker, and put it and the cane in the trunk.

"So you got married on August 27, 1938! Sixty-three years ago today! If that isn't something!"

"Yes."

Then I remember his ailing knees. A week ago I took him to an orthopedic doctor who injected cortisone in each knee. "On a scale of one to ten, how badly do your knees hurt today, Edward?"

"About a six," he says without hesitation.

"A six? That's painful," I frown.

A few minutes later I ease my car into a handicapped parking spot abutting a roofed walkway connecting the parish center building to the church. I hurry around to the passenger side to open the door for him. I pop the trunk and get out the walker and open it. A man approaches whom I recognize.

"Edward, I want you to meet Harvey. He's our music director. Harvey, this is Edward. He's celebrating his sixty-third wedding anniversary today. His wife is home and is bedridden."

"Pleased to meet you," Harvey says, shaking Edward's hand. I'm in his choir and this is the first time I see Harvey wearing shorts. Somehow they don't become him.

Another familiar figure approaches. It's Father Ambrose, our pastor, heading for church to celebrate mass. He's wearing a black suit with a Roman collar.

"Hi, Father Ambrose," I say. "Edward is celebrating his sixty-third wedding anniversary today."

"Yes, I know," he smiles. I wonder how he knows. Edward must have called the parish center office and left word for Father Ambrose to mention the anniversary at mass. We follow Father Ambrose to the side door, and the priest holds the door open for Edward. Father Ambrose's jet-black hair contrasts with Edward's faded black and gray hair. I motion Father Ambrose inside and hold the door for him.

I follow as Edward pushes his walker across the orange-brown carpeting into the second pew near the door. The first two pews by the door are reserved for the handicapped. Edward folds his walker and pushes it to the end of the pew and sits down. I sit down beside him. The dozen or so people already present conclude a rosary: "Holy Mary, mother of God, pray for us sinners, now and at the hour of our death, amen," they repeat.

A few minutes later a tall, blonde altar girl, carrying a lighted candle, precedes Father Ambrose from the sacristy to the sanctuary. He stops at the altar and begins mentioning names of people for whom the mass will be offered. Looking to his left toward Edward, and speaking in a deep voice with a strong foreign accent, he concludes with, " ...and for Edward and Diane on their sixty-third wedding anniversary." I turn to Edward and smile. He beams.

After Father Ambrose concludes his brief homily, about not being afraid to follow God's call, he reads a few petitions and asks the congregation to voice their requests. A woman says, "For my aunt, who is having surgery today, we pray to the Lord." Everyone responds with "Lord, hear our prayer."

After two more petitions are voiced, I speak out, "For Edward and Diane on their sixty-third wedding anniversary." I stop, waiting for people to say, "Lord, hear our prayer," but hear nothing but silence. Then I remember: I am supposed to say, "We pray to the Lord," which I quickly add. Then comes the "Lord, hear our prayer." I'm glad I voice the petition, even though Father Ambrose mentioned Edward's anniversary at the beginning of mass.

When mass is over, several people drift

forward to congratulate Edward and ask about his wife. "She's bedridden and has Alzheimer's. But her vital signs are good," he tells them.

As I follow Edward to the car, he says, "Can you take me to the flower shop? I want to get Diane a bouquet." His eyes sparkle and the corners of his mouth arch into a smile.

"Sure. You mean the shop on the other side of the parking lot?"

"Yes."

I open the door for him and place the folded walker in the trunk. I find a parking place, albeit an illegal one, right next to the side door of the floral shop. I park and hold the door open for Edward as he pushes his walker inside. A bird screeches. I see two cages. Inside one are two large, colorful birds; inside the other are four small, equally colorful birds.

A young woman wearing shorts and blouse approaches. She has on no makeup, and her straight, short, brown hair looks as if it is still wet from a shower.

"Which bird is making all the noise?" I ask.

"The small one," she says with a heavy accent.

"Which small one?" I ask.

"The small one," she repeats. I leave well enough alone. Okay, so it's the small one. I take her word for it. Apparently she doesn't understand my question. Or maybe I don't understand her reply.

"Do you have any carnations?" Edward asks.

"Yes. Only red ones."

"Okay. I'll take twenty-four red carnations and

some baby breath. Can you make them into a bouquet?" He voices the question as though he had asked it many times.

"Yes," she says, and heads for a refrigerated, glassed enclosure and brings out a large container of crimson long-stem carnations. I wonder about their freshness.

"Please, you sit down," she says. "It take me five minutes."

We sit down on a white bench alongside the bird cages. I turn and begin to make soft whistle noises and clicking sounds at one of the large birds.

"He loves the attention," a woman without an accent says from a nearby office.

"What kind of birds are they?" I ask.

"The large ones are cockatiels, and the small ones are canaries."

One of the cockatiels approaches me inside its cage. It is gray with a yellow head. Every time I mouth a sound, it cocks its head and peers at me.

"He's probably wondering why he had never seen a bird without hair on it before," I laughingly comment to Edward, referring to my own baldness. He laughs.

"Which bird is the one that is so loud?" I ask the woman in the office.

"The one you're talking to," she says.

"So you're the noisy guy," I tease. It creeps close to me along the wire cage, pivoting its head back and forth like a metronome.

"Your bouquet ready," the woman with the strong accent says.

349

Edward, clinging to his walker, gets up from the bench and heads for the counter. I follow. The woman with the accent is wrapping the bouquet of carnations and baby breath in a sheet of dark-green paper. She counts the carnations.

"I think I give you twenty-three," she says. "I give you one more." She hurries to the flower compartment and returns with another carnation and inserts it into the bouquet. Edward hands her his Visa credit card.

"I'll take the bouquet out to the car," I tell Edward.

"All right."

I very carefully pick up the wrapped flowers and carry the precious cargo to the car, setting it ever so gently on the back seat. I return to the shop, and Edward is half way to the door. I hold it open for him, watching him push his walker up a slight incline. I open the car door for him and put his walker in the trunk.

Back at Edward's house, the nurse's aide's car is gone, so I back into the driveway. I get the walker and cane out of the trunk, open the car door for him, spread open the walker, and hang his cane over the iron railing leading up to the porch.

The melodious song of a scarlet cardinal draws my eyes to Edward's chimney. "Look, Edward, a cardinal is perched on your TV antenna and singing you an anniversary song! Isn't that something, huh!"

Edward stops and, clutching his walker, strains to look up. "Yes, that is something." His handsome features melt into a smile.

"I'll take the bouquet into the house. Where would you like me to put it?" I know it would be inappropriate for me to give it to Diane.

"Put it on the dining room table," Edward says. I hurry inside, deposit the bouquet on the table, and go back outside. Edward leaves the walker at the railing and uses his cane as an aid in getting up the steps to the porch. I close my car doors and the trunk lid, fold the walker, and follow him inside.

"May I hang up your coat for you?" I ask after depositing the walker in the vestibule.

"Yes," he says, taking it off and handing it to me. I put it on a hanger and return it to the closet.

At the top of the vestibule steps, Edward places his cane on the console and switches to his inside-the-house walker. This walker is equipped with a black pouch for his personal items. I feel a stir of excitement as he heads for the dining room table and the bouquet.

He stops at the table. "May I carry the bouquet for you?" I ask.

"Yes."

I pick it up and follow Edward as he pushes his walker toward Diane. He stops at the bed and looks lovingly at his wife. She's lying on her back, and the head of the bed tilts up at about a 30-degree angle. Diane's wan face with small features and blue eyes looks straight ahead, showing no sign of cognition. Her snow-white hair is nicely combed. A white, silk nightgown and white blanket cover her gaunt figure. I hand the bouquet to Edward, and he takes it and places it across Diane's chest, with the open end of the bouquet on her left.

I suddenly recall speaking briefly with Diane three years earlier in church. Dorothy, my wife, and I were leaving the 5 o'clock mass when she introduced me to Diane and Edward, whom Dorothy got to know from attending the daily 8:30 morning mass. Diane was walking very erect next to Edward, who was bent over pushing a walker.

"They just celebrated their sixtieth wedding anniversary," Dorothy said.

Something prompted me to ask Diane, "What is the most important element in a successful marriage?"

"You have to be in love," she said matter-of-factly, following her husband out the church side door.

"Oh," I smiled, reflecting on her reply. I have thought about the wisdom of those words many times since.

"Happy sixty-third wedding anniversary, darling," Edward says softly. How handsome he is, even at 89, I remind myself. My eyes glaze over. Diane continues to look straight ahead, but her lips quaver as she mumbles something. Her right hand edges up and her fingers travel slowly around the green paper. Her left hand remains under her blanket.

"May I turn the bouquet around so her right hand can feel the flowers?" I ask Edward.

"Yes."

I gently lift the bouquet and turn it around so the flowers are on her right side. Her right hand begins to caress the carnations, like a mother running her fingers over the face of her baby. The carnations appear to be freshly cut. She continues to mumble something unintelligible. Do I imagine that the corners of her mouth lift into a slight smile? I take out my handkerchief and wipe my eyes.

"Are you happy, darling?" Edward asks lovingly. Diane continues to mumble and caress the flowers and look straight ahead. I dab my eyes again.

I glance at Marina, standing nearby watching. Her eyes, too, are moist.

"Edward, I think I ought to be leaving. You say you don't need me for any errands this week?"

"No."

"Okay. Then I'll be seeing you at four-thirty Saturday for the five-o'clock mass. If you need me before then, don't hesitate to give me a call."

"All right. And thanks, Joe." His eyes effervesce.

"It was my pleasure." I head out to my car, wiping my eyes.

CPSIA information can be obtained at www.ICGtesting.com
Printed in the USA
LVOW041540010712

288408LV00001B/147/P